# GLOBAL ATHLETES BIBLE

## NOTE

This volume was initially conceived as a simple survey of the nutritional supplementary aids energizing athletic performance. Soon however, our inquiry grew into a challenging project involving a study of various athletes who have used vitamin/mineral supplementation to significantly expand their athletic horizons.

*At no time do we pretend to be diagnostic or perscriptive in the following chapters.* Such tasks are best left to your physician. But, we certainly do hope to be educational, provocative, and interesting.

In *ALL* cases where dosage recommendations appear, they have been worked up to after extended periods of training and must be read in that context. Above all, be critical and understand the contents.

GLOBAL HEALTH LTD.
BOX 18, SITE 1, RR2
TOFIELD, ALBERTA, CANADA
TOB 4J0

ISBN - 0-921202-01-6

P9-DWO-356

# GLOBAL ATHLETES BIBLE

## DEAR READER

This book was built as a result of the knowledge and efforts of many individuals, who have brought varied background and areas of expertise to the field of athletic nutrition and supplementation. Their collaboration has given rise to a unique approach and style, which we at Global Health believe will go a long way towards educating the health conscious public about natural nutritional supplementation at the level of athletic performance, and fitness in general.

The health and fitness industry today is more alive with changes, challenges and choices than at any other period in history. We at Global, trust that this work will adequately reflect and explain the existing dynamism. Regardless of your partricular athletic endeavour this book will certainly expand your overall awareness on athletic nutrition, as well as familiarize you with your own special needs in this area.

Our readers will find this work rather timely, particularly in the context of the current international campaign against the

# GLOBAL ATHLETES BIBLE

use of various stimulants in high level athletic performance and competition. In this respect, we are all united in our commitment to contribute towards the development of safe and natural alternatives.

With this in mind, Global Health wishes to acknowledge the following contributors towards this interesting collective effort.

| | |
|---|---|
| **Global Health Ltd.** | **Text Design** |
| **Betty Gervais** | **Computing** |
| **Kathy Kesslar** | **Global Assistant** |
| **Evelyn Stevens** | **"          "** |
| **Fred Thompson** | **Special Advise** |
| **Mikael Taffesse** | **"          "** |
| **Phil Brunner** | **"          "** |
| **Sandra Nyholt** | **"          "** |
| **Azeb Zemarian** | **"          "** |

**Photography**
**by**
**Zinger Photographics Ltd.**

# GLOBAL ATHLETES BIBLE

# TABLE OF CONTENTS

# GLOBAL ATHLETES BIBLE

## DEDICATION

All health and fitness conscious individauls can benefit from the nutritional and supplemental principles ellaborated and illustrated in the following pages. We think it is possible to be fit and stay healthy throughout life, but only when one understands the general laws governing nutrition and supplementation.

This book is particularly dedicated to those rare disciplined beings throughout the world, who tirelessly and unceasingly seek to achieve excellence in their athletic endeavours. Without a reflection on the contemporary issues explored in these pages, serious athletes could put themselves at a severe disadvantage in todays perfection oriented, and drug-testing competitive world of sports. In the final analysis, this book is dedicated to all athletes, past, present, and future.

We know that this volume will generate significant controversy in many quarters. We do not only welcome this, but it is one of the risks we are prepared to assume in order to advance our knowledge of physical culture freely and daringly. As in all areas of life, authorities and experts in the field of health and nutrition also hold divergent views and approaches concerning athletic performance. Ours is the Global way!

# GLOBAL ATHLETES BIBLE

## FORWORD

People are paying a lot more attention these days to physical fitness, and, therefore more interest on the possibilities of a healthy, vigorous and productive life in an increasingly hazardous world.

In fact, according to Stats Canada, "participation by Canadians in physical activity has increased seven fold since 1972. An estimated 11.6 million Canadians aged 10 or older, representing 56% of the population, are now regarded as active-devoting at least three hours a week to exercise...." (Globe and Mail Wed Sept 9, 1987.)

This phenomenon is global and represents a clear indication of the influence and sweep of the fitness revolution, at least in the North American context. For this fitness revolution to have a more lasting and fundamental effect however, it is our belief and recommendation that the practice of balanced nutrition and proper supplementation should be an indispensable part of the three hours already devoted to physical exercise. Apart from the obvious mental and physical benefits, the long term effect may well be a vast improvement in the health, and athletic abilities of the population at large. Today both medicine and competitive sports are costly and complicated businesses. Nutritional supplementation is the key for high-level fitness and health today.

The athletic community in which we partake, is rapidly making headway in this nutrition conscious direction. Informed by the latest findings in bio-chemistry and the services of an impressive array of high-tech precision instruments.

Sports nutrition is coming of age. Research has conclusively demonstrated that the champions way is through the scientific use of vitamin-mineral supplements and nutritional concentrates, to effectively boost his/her energy. While the amount of scientific knowledge in this area is rapidly expanding, most athletes are ill-equiped to understand the increasingly esoteric language and decipher the controversies arising from the different schools of thought on this subject. Nor can they afford the services of a professional performance nutritionist. Most M. D.'s curriculums are also sadly deficient in this respect. This reality not only places the majority of aspiring athletes at a competitive disadvantage, but renders them susceptible to misinformation, and the illicit "performance drugs" currently being peddled by charlatan "gurus" and assorted profiteers and pharmaceutical salesmen so prevelent around todays gyms and fitness clubs.  This trend needs to be reversed.

Sports scientists and elite-level competitors know one thing for certain. Namely, all things being more or less equal the athlete who makes   superior gain in strength and acquires greater  development in the necessary mental and physical skills, is the one competently   informed by modern nutritional techniques.   Thus, in an intensely competitive world where fractions of a second, and one more last rep make all the difference, knowledge in this area is becoming vitally important for developing athletes and coaches alike.   We live in an athletic environment where close to a dozen world records in as many track and field events, are set and shattered.   In light of B. Johnson's historic performance, the 10 second barrier for the 100 meter appears prehistoric, pushing the limits of man's athletic ability and potentials even further.

Our task in this volume is to make the

state- of-the-art information available to all athletes in a concise and intelligible form without sacrificing content. This project is part of our ongoing commitment to train athletes and performers on how to start understanding and supplementing their energy intake for maximum performance in their own chosen athletic endeavours. Flooded with pollutants, drugs, and additives in our food, air, and water, we all owe it to ourselves to know as much as possible about what we ingest. This is very fundamental to the pursuit of life. It is our sincerest hope therefore, that this volume will be your companion in your ongoing quest for athletic excellence and total fitness. The information contained in the following pages will certainly change your approach to training, and health in general.

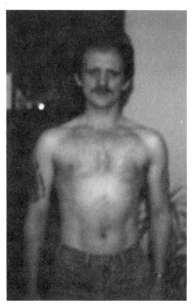 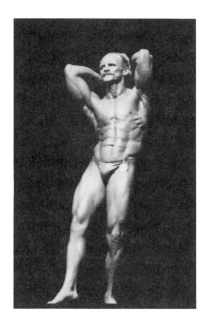

**Before**                    **After**

## HEALTH, NUTRITION & SUPPLEMENTATION TODAY

More than the population at large, improving their health is particularly important to all athletes and even greater among competitive athletes. They are well aware that in todays intensely competitive world, their potentials for optimum performance are based on maximum health, which in our mind is largely based on proper nutrition and supplementation. Perhaps we are reflecting the athlete's bias in our

thoughts,
but the fitness lifestyle as a whole, is the surest and most accessible way of preserving and improving our health in the fashion envisioned by the WHO. That is a perspective more oriented towards well being and health, as opposed to disease and surgery. Physical exercise does strengthen the heart, lungs, and circulation, while also toning our entire musculo-skeletal system. To our way of thinking, a truly healthy lifestyle is impossible without regular physical exercise and proper nutrition. Scientifically speaking, diet is one of the most important indicators on how long and active an individual's life will be.

Scientific studies have repeatedly shown that active people do enjoy better health and live longer and more productively than sedentary people. By choosing the fitness lifestyle, North Americans have clearly demonstrated that they too, no longer subscribe to the idea that the mere "absence of disease" is indicative of a healthy state of existence in todays inherently stressful society, Stress too, daily robs the body of energy and substances by depleting the body of vitamins and minerals, thereby significantly reducing physical and mental efficiency. Once aware that they all activate the same brain receptors however, we would rather be fortified and supplemented by the nutrients INOSITOL and NIACINAMIDE today, than be on Valium for any period of time. This outmoded approach to health bears some serious rethinking. The maintenance of optimum health is literally the business of the competitive athlete. In brief, be as healthy as you possibly can. Every aspiring athlete would be well advised to think likewise. Just as we need physical activity we also must have adequate nutrition to protect against health risks in todays society.

In our experience as a nutritional consulting team, we can unequivocally say, that from a survey of the common health problems for which people approach us, most are rooted in the nutritional habits and lifestyles of the individuals. Despite modern discoveries in the nutritional and sports sciences, and the apparent all around affluence, it is our experience that a pervasive form of malnutrition prevails in our societies today. In our opinion, most severe diseases today (cancer, heart attacks) etc., can be clearly linked to dietary ignorance and lack of physical culture.

It is a malnutrition not so much based on the lack of basic food products, but more due to the ignorant consumption of foods and chemical substances which have been proven detrimental to human health explicitly and implicitly. It is high time that we realize this and accept responsibilty for our health, and act by modifying our lifestyles to minimize the hazards caused by chemicalized diets. Athletic people particularly, recognize that they require specific nutrients in qualities that can no longer be readily furnished through a "fork and knife" approach to diet, in today's world. It is a lifestyle worth learning from.

Our environment today has become degraded and poisoned by pollutants, toxins, additive chemicals and assorted insecticides, seriously depleting the quality of most readily available overprocessed food products in the stores. Simply avoiding the cummulative effects of these degraded nutrients, should necessitate the regular use of modern nutritional techniques and supplementation. Still, widespread vitamin and mineral deficiencies are serious health problems today. Without adequate supplemental fortification these deficiency problems are certain to arise.

According to the U.S. department of Agriculture, close to 2/3 of Americans are deficient in one or more essential vitamins and minerals. In the wake of the ecological ravages caused by the modern industrial revolution, the search for alternative sources of natural nutrients has also come a long way. Since the vitamin was first discovered in 1913, scientists have isolated some forty vitamins and minerals that effect every aspect of our neuro-physical process. Vitamins are intimately involved in all our metabolic processes. Simply put, vitamins are catalysts which assist in the digestion and absorption of nutrients in our system. Their absence, hampers the efficient utilization of nutrients thereby minimizing our resistance to stress and premature aging. As coenzymes, they play an important biochemical role by participating in the synthesis of energy for athletic activity. Their deficiency significantly reduces the functional and tissue repair capacities of all our organs, seriously effecting our energy and health levels. The quality of the nutrition or a diet is put to test, particularly when we are under heavy physical or emotional stress.

Boosting athletic performance and sports endurance through the use of vitamin-mineral supplements is a new and exciting area of research today. It is also in this context that sports nutrition and supplementation is fast maturing into a science and art onto itself.

Athletic performance has been one of mankind's greatest preoccupations in every culture since the first recorded classic Olympic Games in 776 BC. Sufficient documents exist to confirm that the relationship between nutrition and performance was as much a central preoccupation with the ancient Olympians and their coaches, as with present day champions and their trainers. These days however, there is much more at stake with olympic victories, than the olive wreaths bestowed on the ancient champions. Literally millions of dollars in prizes, endorsements and media appearances, await those rare athletes who achieve optimum performance.

Although the dessicated heart of the lion and the testicles of other powerful animals might not be included in the modern athletic nutritionists therapeutic practices, the search for ergogenic foods (those that enhance the capacity for physical or mental labour), continues unabetted, only with much more practical scientific applications today. Todays nutritional supplements are widely recognized as a safe, scientific way to ensure health, prevent nutritional disorders, to increase immune responses, and raise levels of athletic performance considerably. World class trainers and professional athletes make use of this valuable knowledge, and the possibilities are limitless. They know full well, that through the proper coordination and manipulation of nutrients, the functional capacity of every organ can be somewhat restored and enhanced.

While every potential athlete cannot be expected to follow up on the latest nutritional discoveries vis-a-vis the sports sciences, it is his/her responsibility to, at least "understand" the critical role nutrients and supplements play in their conditioning process as well as developement into healthy athletes and human beings. Our own methods of training athletes are closely anchored in these simple holistic considerations.

# GLOBAL ATHLETES BIBLE

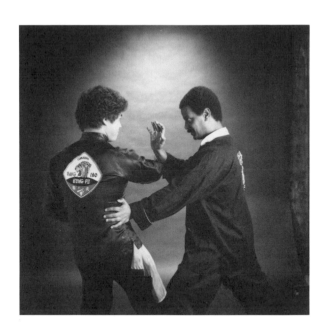

### *PERSONALIZED COUNSELLING*

Based on this background, when interested athletes approach us, the first consultation is structured around the elimination of their degenerative lifestyle traits, at least from the nutritional angle. Alcohol too, is a great vitamin depleter. It is no longer enough to state that everyone needs adequate supplies of carbohydrates, fat, protein, vitamins, minerals and beverages. From the performance point of view, an athlete's need is far more proportionate, delicate and complex. For starters, an athlete needs extra calories just to maintain ideal body weight while training. Nutrient needs do change from one athlete to the next, depending on many variables including gender. Thus, this first consultation also enables us to begin structuring a corrective nutritional plan designed to help the athlete achieve his/her distinct personal athletic goals fast, *NATURALLY*, and successfully. For our subsequent meeting, the athlete is requested to write down *literally everything* that goes into his/her mouth for the next three days and advised to see a physician for a general check up.

In the course of our next exchange, we hope to make the athlete *nutrition-conscious,* based on the list he or she submitted. That is, we try to enlighten them about the impact of diet on performance and quality of health. If severe nutritional deficiencies are detected, the person is placed on a form of nutrition and health therapy to restore proper metabolic balance, before a suitable training program is outlined. Every serious athlete, bodybuilder, or weight trainer interested in raising his/her performance level, will benefit from this approach. Any successful nutritional program must be individualized, and designed according to the bio-chemical and mechanical characteristics of the individual athlete and his/her objectives. A simplified trendy diet is a rather poor substitute, if one at all.

During this phase we rely heavily on vitamins (organic molecules), minerals (inorganic molecules), amino acids, and generally proper nutrition, to provide the individual with his/her daily balanced caloric needs necessary to safely achieve the desired athletic objective. The actual calculations, nutrient choices and balance, are tedious and thorough. We point to the research evidence, and our own experiences, that the many natural supplements we recommend will significantly help them in their efforts to achieve their desired weight and obtain increased athletic capabilities, *we strongly warn, that in themselves, supplements are worth very little.* They only work in tandem with a healthy diet and sensible lifestyle to keep the body running efficiently and at its best capacity. They truly ensure, and effectively supplement our own committments to athletic excellence, training, and superior health. In other words, they are truly ergogenic and especially necessary for the serious athlete. For any athlete over thirty they are simply indispensible. This point will be highlighted in due course. For now, let it be said that a planned nutritional and training program, aided by supplementation, is strongly recommended to enhance health and performance all around.

*No fad diets of whatever kind can be depended upon* in the long run because they tend to be radically imbalanced. Basically, what you eat determines your energy and performance level. Junk foods merely drain the alkaline from your body, resulting in serious loss of several essential nutrients.

It is also our practice and experience that "high octane" or quality nutrients and supplements (vitamins, minerals, amino acids, trace elements) etc., when administered in the proper dosage and ratio, can authentically be relied upon to restore health and enhance the body's ability to convert energy into performance. Scientists have not only isolated the exact hormone known as *"growth hormone"* in the pituitary gland, but have also discovered how to trigger our body's release of this hormone through natural amino acids that are safe, and for the most part available in every Health Food Store without perscription.

In recent years the restorative healing powers of protein amino acid supplements have been the subject of many interesting clinical researches. In post surgery recoveries, alcohol and drug addictions, stress related deficiencies, allergies, cancer cases etc., protein amino-acids have been experimentally proven to aid and accelerate the healing process and decrease the aging process as well.

Athletically speaking, the body requires certain conditions to function optimally, fundamental of which is a sound health. To our mind, the essential precondition can be gained and maintained with a program where advanced nutritional techniques with properly formulated supplementations, play a leading part. In our own practice we have seen and recorded phenomenal successes with our students and the different athletes we have had occasion to design nutritional therapy for (short and long distance runners, martial artists, bodybuilders, professional dancers) etc. They have all reported an enhanced sense of well-being (Psychopharmacological effects) and a marked improvement in their own chosen athletic endeavour, upon administration of various amino acids such as *L-ORNITHINE , L-ARGININE, TRYPTOPHAN, METHIONINE* , etc.

In this process, the psychological dimensions of commitment, self-discipline, mental conditioning etc., must not be lost sight of. A sense of trust must be instilled between trainer and athlete. we try to assure our students that we can increase their energy, stamina, endurance, and improve their physique, only with their full cooperation and participation. Nutritional therapy simply put, involves getting the athletes to eat right, help them gain weight or stop the weight loss whatever the case may be, and nutritionally prepare their bodies for higher performance capacities. The record clearly shows that those athletes who consistently and fully follow their program and instructions, have also managed to excell in their performance levels.

Our own initiation to the athletic world started relatively late in life, and was largely made possible by very strict nutritional guidelines. Approximately 80% of our success can be attributed to effective nutritional practices. More so than any other athlete, the signs of inadequate nutrition are immediately visible on a competing  bodybuilder's physique as opposed to say, a martial artist or a wrestler. To be sure, the latter's performance would also surely deteriorate in later rounds on account of the same problem, ie. fatigue and exhaustion will result due to nutritional deficiencies. The fate of every athlete depends on the combination and quality of the nutrients that fuel his energy to accomplish the task.

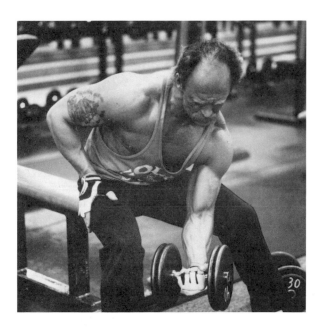

# GLOBAL ATHLETES BIBLE

## *WEIGHT & RESISTANCE TRAINING FOR PEAK PERFORMANCE*

Once on a sound nutritional path, a resistance training program can be embarked upon for outstanding results in health, body shaping and overall improved performance, It is our belief that resistance training helps elevate performance in other sports, and in this respect the empirical evidence has also proved very encouraging.

Most athletes who approach us for weight training tips and programs do not usually want to be bodybuilders in the fullest sense of the term. Instead, they're interested in using our expertise to help them strengthen and define their bodies, build mass and/or strength in the important muscle groups and generally improve the lean muscle to fat ratio of their bodies. They come from all areas of the sports world, and are aware that in athletic performance the problem is not really bodyweight, but rather bodyfat. In this respect, say a marathon runner and a gymnast have different nutritional needs than a line-backer and a boxer, but both are interested in gaining pure muscle mass and strength, while reducing their body fat which restricts peak performance, in all athletic endeavours. Here, nutritional knowhow provides the edge.

**Our advice and practice in this area consists of:**

**1. Conditioning and strengthening the body as a whole.**

**2. Strengthening the main muscles and connective tissue involved in their chosen activity.**

**3. Achieving a muscle-balance between the extensor and flexor muscles.**

**4. Going with them through some developemental weight exercises that promote general health, strength, and what we call muscle- consciousness, with emphasis on developing their underdeveloped muscle groups.**

In the final analysis, our system is really no different than other qualified nutrition consultants, except for our approach. Namely, resistance training plays a great part in our system of enhancing performance and health.

# GLOBAL ATHLETES BIBLE

Our emphasis is on isotension, resistance, and generally using accurate techniques that set in motion maximum amounts of muscle fibres and cells with slower but lighter, more intense movements. Throughout the motion, we encourage the athletes to concentrate deeply on the feeling inside the muscles, instead of on the weights. It is no longer a secret that weight training is not only a factor in ultimate performance, but it's the foundation that helps many world-class athletes (including Ben Johnson), hold their lead or edge, whatever the case may be.

Resistance training, is a vitally important component of our system. Aside from the technicalities involved, we try to counsel our students on the most efficient way to burn fat while gaining the necessary muscle mass and strength, and by introducing them to the appropriate amino acids considered to be *GH (growth hormone)* releasers. Some amino acids are especially suited for burning fat while building muscles. In this respect the amino acids *L-TYROSINE, L-TRYPTOPHAN, L-ARGININE, L-LYSINE, L-ORNITHINE, L-METHIONINE, L-CARNITINE, and L-GLYCINE,* come to mind as extremely potent and valuable sports performance nutrients, when coordinated with a well balanced diet and workout program. Anybody engaged in a regular athletic or exercise program can benefit significantly from proper diet and supplementation. Whatever the case, the method of supplemental amino acid use is very important in achieving the desired objectives in todays athletic world.

A combination of exercise, diet, and supplementation, can improve your lean muscle to fat ratio, accelerate your circulatory-metabolic process and significantly help your progress towards fitness and good health, while providing immunity to many illnesses. *GH* releasing amino acids like *ARGININE* etc., in and of themselves, will not result in any noticeable muscle growth, while they are very effective in maintaining your muscle gains and definition during the off season. In this context, we have found that the nutrient supplements *CHOLINE and VITAMIN B5* when taken together in a *ratio of 3:1*, are very helpful in maintaining muscle tone and definition, with the minimum of exercise. Among its other uses *CHOLINE* is essential for the proper utilization of fatty foods, with *VITAMIN B5 OR PANTOTHENIC ACID,* making this function possible. *VITAMIN B5* is also essential for the synthesis of fat and sugar to energy, and vital to the integrity of our adrenal glands and our central nervous system.

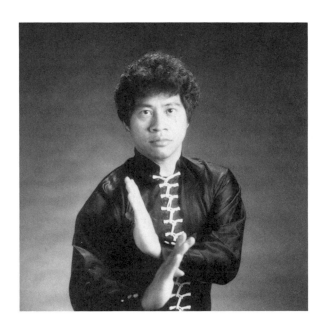

# GLOBAL ATHLETES BIBLE

## CARBOHYDRATES

*Carbohydrates, or "carbs"*, are extremely important for everyday life sustaining neuro-physical functions and the athletes principal source of energy. In addition to the more obvious daily physical needs, the brain almost exclusively relies on carbs for energy. Thus, a diet deficient in carbs is sure to result in somewhat lower levels of mental and physical efficiency. In the sedentary person this may cause potential health problems. If you are an athlete however, this situation becomes rather critical, as it impinges on your performance capacity as a whole. In short, carbohydrates are an absolutely necessary nutritional requirement for proper body and mental functioning.

In terms of chemistry, carbohydrates are composed of carbon, hydrogen, and oxygen molecules, and except for glycogen, lactic acid and ribose, most carbs are of plant origin. *Carbohydrates contain approximately 4 calories per gram* the same as protein, but are primarily composed of starches and sugars. At rest, about 35% of the muscle's fuel is contributed by carbohydrates (glycogen and glucose), and the remainder (the majority), by fats. When the athlete starts performing at peak level however, glycogen begins to provide up to 90% of the necessary muscle's fuel. Towards the end, or during the later phases in say, a triathelon, fats begin to provide larger and larger percentages of our energy needs.

Nutritionists conveniently classify carbohydrates as simple and complex, depending on their nutritional qualities. In this manner, grains, legumes, and all sorts of vegetables are classified as complex carbohydrates, while sucrose based products, like your ordinary chocolate bar or candies, are classified as simple carbohydrates. The distinction for our purposes, lies in the different nutritional chemical elements they provide to fuel the athlete's mental and physical capacity. The latter carbohydrates in our mind, have neither nutritional nor *ergogenic* (performance enhancing) qualities except in the very temporary and negative sense. Once absorbed, sucrose rapidly agitates blood sugar rise, heightening release of insulin and hence the conversion of sucrose to body fat and even possible hypoglycemia in the long run. If you consume more calories than you need, insulin strongly stimulates fat storage. Of late, the chemical combination of the two amino acids *PHENYLALANINE and ASPARTIC ACID* have given rise to various alternate products, whose virtues lie in not percipititating this dangerous increase in blood sugar level. Incidentally, carbohydrate foods also activate the levels of *PHENYLALANINE* in the brain.

Because of the extreme physical and mental demands experienced by athletes during regular training and competition, their nutritional needs as a group vary significantly from non-athletic or average people. This is rather fundamental. Athletes not only expend different types and amounts of energy, but also experience high levels of physical and mental stress in a competitive situation. Athletes are continually restructuring their metabolic process in training, and are known to have 25% higher glycogen storage capabilities.

*GLYCOGEN*, which is the word used to describe our reserves of carbohydrates, is primarily stored in the different muscle tissues, where it becomes the most readily available source of athletic energy. Upon consumption of complex carbs, they are absorbed into the small intestine and enzymatically regulated throughout our musculo-skeletal system. Knowledge of the particular dynamics of glycogen storage in our system, is vitally important for any athlete who strives to obtain higher levels of physical efficiency and performance capacity. Simply put, *GLYCOGEN* in the muscles and liver, and *GLUCOSE* in the blood are the determining sources of energy for hard, demanding and intense exercises or workouts.

Many world-class athletes (cyclists, long distance runners, bodybuilders) etc., have for long periods manipulated their glycogen storage in the hopes of elevating their energy into greater stamina, strength and endurance levels. Performance gains through glucose polymers are now well documented facts. The level of physical activity and performance among todays triathelon super-performance athletes is truly awesome. Sports scientists and coaches have been known to dramatically increase athletic endurance by administering and adjusting carbohydrate intake in such competitions. A definite index of insufficient complex carbohydrate intake in our diet is the premature onset of exhaustion throughout the body. The type and timing factor in your carb diet will at this point decidedly regulate your athletic fate. Athletes make use of this fact to increase development and progress in their physical capacity. Sufficient glycogen storage then, is indespensible for hard, extended training loads and superior performance. Scientists estimate that to continue exercising at this level of intensity, muscle glycogen has to be maintained *above 4 mg per kilogram* of bodyweight. Thus, an adequate understanding of the precise effects of carbohydrates is a key to authentic supremacy in todays sports world.

At this stage, the main concern for the athlete is that he/she receive the appropriate amounts and types of carbohydrates necessary for his/her specific sport, without exceeding caloric needs. When this occurs successfully, the athlete will not only be able to increase his/her capacity, but he/she will also be able to maintain ideal body weight. This is much like walking a proverbial razor blade. It is a highly important athletic principle. If the body absorbs more carbohydrates than necessary for its glucose supply in the blood, and glycogen storage in the liver, the surplus is stored either in the form of body fat, or utilized to fuel exercise and training. In terms of performance, although in ample supply, *bodyfat is the last and least efficient source of energy!* Our systems resort to this energy source only when glycogen is totally depleted. In terms of aesthetics, the consequences are equally disasterous. Maintenance of bodyweight therefore, is very important in the manipulation of nutrients for optimal performance capacity. Whether one has a surplus of fat tissue or not, is quite symptomatic of their level of fitness in terms of athletics.

Although averages do not take specific physiological and metabolic conditions into consideration, anywhere from *1/2 to 2/3 of a competitive athletes daily caloric intake should come from carbohydrates,* strictly depending of course, on the specific charactaristics of the individual, and the sport involved. In short, carbohydrate needs vary with the type of athletic training and intensity. For example, if you are an endurance athlete and primarily seek to activate your aerobic energy, you should compensate by increasing your intake of specific complex carbohydrates. Football is largely based on the use of anaerobic metabolism, both cycling and swimming tend to utilize aerobic metabolism over-whelmingly. Different sports have different energy requirements that can be complemented and boosted by appropriate nutritional guidelines and techniques.

To be sure, all carbohydrates will produce some kind of energy. *But the quality of the carbohydrate and the timing of consumption will defenitely determine the quality of your athletic performance.* as in the triathelon scenario alluded to earlier. To adequately understand this point, it is necessary to take a look into the ways our body absorbs, metabolizes and utilizes its carbohydrate intake.

The conversion of nutrients into energy starts with the carbohydrates we consume. The body assimilates and synthesizes the different qualities of carbohydrates differently and at different rates into the bloodstream. Nutritionists calculate this rate by what is known as the *GLYCEMIC INDEX.* which simply measures the relative glucose effect of foods. *In performance terms, the lower the glycemic rating, the longer lasting and more consistent the energy provided.* For example, apples are rated less than bananas, oats less than cornflakes, peanuts less than potatochips etc.. The complex carbohydrates are generally rated less than the simple ones, although there are some rare and important exceptions. Thus, not all complex carbs provide long term energy. Always, as a rule of thumb, replace high-glycemic-index carbohydrates in your diet with low-glycemic-index carbohydrates, and increase fibre consumption. At about 3 grams daily, it will also significantly slow the absorption of carbohydrates in food, thereby decreasing their effective glycemic index. This indexing can easily be verified by references to various sports nutritional and medical charts and guides, and needs no reproduction here. The point we are trying to get across here, is that the quality and balance of the necessary complex carbohydrate intake can be precisely monitored by calculating the aerobic and anaerobic components and demands of your particular athletic endeavour. All athletic endeavours require a blend of both aerobic and anaerobic metabolism.

To be sure, the question of timing your carbohydrate intake also assumes great importance in maximizing your athletic potential through carbohydrate manipulation.

# GLOBAL ATHLETES BIBLE

The rate of glycogen utilization is closely tied to the biochemistry of our body, and is best explained in that context. We have already stated, that the simple sucrose varieties of the carbohydrates are best deleted from the athletes menu, because of their negative impact on the overall metabolic process. A few hardcore weightlifters may disagree with this. Still, their direct rush through the bloodstream temporarily causes havoc in our blood sugar levels, that is really not conducive for extended optimum energy. This temporary rush in energy merely causes insulin reaction, and an inevitable drastic reduction in energy 1/2 hour later. Thus, for our purpose, the relevent glycogen can only come from the complex variety.

To be sure, if sufficient supply of carbohydrate is not available to meet the athletes demand for energy, then amino acids from muscle and other tissues can also be broken down and synthesized to meet this energy demand. This is debilitating and unhealthy to the athlete. We'll learn more about protein dynamics in the chapters ahead. One of the principal features of dietary carbs, is what is known as their "protein-sparing" action, ie., by supplying the necessary energy, they restore protein to its particular and proper functions. The point here, is that the absence of the requisite carbs in our diet can ultimately cause the progressive deterioration of physical and mental functions.

Sports scientists involved in this area, have managed to repeatedly maintain higher glycogen levels, by providing small portions of complex carbs before, during, and after severely demanding workouts. The fifteen minute interval between the portions coincides with the approximate amount of time it takes any strenuous workout to deplete the local muscle glycogen supplies to exhaustion. The athletic fraternity makes good use of these interesting experiments. Runners, weight lifters, swimmers, martial artists, etc., all experience the meaning of this in their daily workouts. Having made this point, the dynamics of athletic carbohydrate utilization may be presented as follows.

Unlike the simple varieties, complex carbohydrates are assimilated into the bloodstream over a period of several hours and utilized accordingly. Unlike fat, which accounts for the vast majority (or 4/5) of the body's energy storage, glycogen is limited in supply and regulated by enzymes that balance its storage in the liver. Aside from converting glycogen from carbs, the liver can also convert blood sugar to free fatty acids and what are known as triglycerides, and distribute them throughout the body either for storage or energy. Theoretically, hard training, elite athletes (endurance runners, bodybuilders, cyclists, boxers) etc., may totally deplete their glycogen stores within an hour or two of moderate to intense exertion and collapse from fatigue caused by total glycogen exhaustion. The symptoms overwhelm the entire body with fatigue, and a lack of coordination of physical functions and skills becomes pronounced. At this level of endurance fatty acids also assume their role as alternate sources of energy.

By the same token, individual muscle groups subjected to intense levels of exercise may use up their own local muscle glycogen supplies (in the muscle tissue) in up to a maximum of 15 minutes. After depletion of their own local sources however, they must revert to the glycogen storage in the liver, which is a considerable source of athletic energy in its own right. As well as glycogen, the liver also converts protein and fat to blood sugar. This transition from one energy source to another is critical, and familiar to all athletes.

To be sure, muscle glycogen is the body's main source of energy for moderate to intense activities of short duration (anaerobic metabolism). During this period, muscle uses proportionate amounts of carbs and fat for energy. But, as the level and duration of exercise intensfies, the muscles "prefer" to depend more on carbs and oxygen because they provide a more efficient energy synthesis. As the triathlon continues, fat contributes an increasingly larger percentage of our energy needs. Depending on its overall development, muscle comprises approximately 40% of the athlete's bodyweight, and uses a proportionate amount of the body's energy even at rest. During high intensity action however, its energy demands increase dramatically and thus, also its need to tap into alternate more efficient energy sources. During these critical periods of transition, the athlete's performance will be seriously undermined and compromised by the lack of appropriate nutritional carbohydrates to fuel and energize the system. It is a veritable struggle between fatigue and victory, "hitting the wall" or successfully tapping into alternative energy sources.

In the latter process, every muscle responds more fluidly and rythmically, pushing ever back the limits of endurance and stamina necessary to accomplish the tasks ahead. This is the privillege of the elite athlete, who has scientifically coordinated his/her carbs with valuable nutritional supplementation in his/her daily training routines and exercises.

The various specialized principles on carbohydrate loading simply extend this dynamic understanding of carbohydrate metabolism further, and attempt to make it applicable to their own sport. The principle involves depleting the muscles glycogen stores completely approximately a week before an important competition, through a combination of totally taxing workouts and dietary manipulation. The first three days require you to abstain from carbs in favour of protein and fats. For the next three days however, you saturate your body with a high carbohydrate diet for which it should be craving. At the time of the event this technique should result in highly supercharged muscles, and increased glycogen storage. The trick consists in nutritionally manipulating the body to store more energy than it ordinarily would. Of course the timing factor varies from individual to individual, but many world class athletes, in different areas have reported increased muscle fluidity and overall increased capacity with the proper application of this rather specialized principle of performance. Bodybuilders too, have their own applications of the carbohydrate loading prinicple.

By following these basic principles, you'll be able to formulate a sound nutritional guideline for maximum performance. When combined with the proper amino acids, and relevant supplements, complex carbs offer the contemporary athlete the proper nutritional fuel for rapidly increasing his/her performance quality. Remember the body places its need for energy above every other need.

# GLOBAL ATHLETES BIBLE

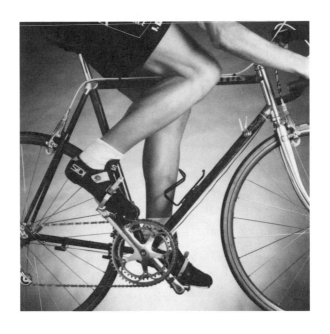

## *SUPPLEMENTARY GUIDE*

Oxygen and nutrients are efficiently carried to every organ and tissue, not only during workouts but also in daily living, as a result of the right nutrients and mineral supplements taken at the appropriate time and in the proper dosage. Human beings are very complex creatures. Approximately eighteen minerals are also known to be required to assure proper regulatory functions and physical maintenance.

In the athletic context, recent studies have indicated that *L-CARNITINE* and *NIACIN* supplementation very significantly enhance performance levels, particularly for athletes who participate in vigorous endurance training and sports. *NIACIN* *(B3)* is intimately involved in the release of energy from carbs, protein, and fats. Like *VITAMIN E,* it is also involved in the dilation of the blood vessels, and the formation of enzymes. This nutrient improves circulation and depresses blood cholestoral levels. *At about a gram daily, that is at levels considerably higher than the Recommended Daily Allowance (RDA),* it has proved to be a vital egrogenic nutrient in our own athletic pursuits. *A word of caution here, begin NIACIN dosage at apporximately 100 mg daily, or less, and increase slowly.* In the area of enhàncing endurance oriented athletic performance *L-CARNITINE and NIACIN* (Nicotinic Acid) have of late attracted considerable attention. Both are produced in the body by amino acids, with *NIACIN* being manufactured from the body by *TRYPTOPHAN. L-CARNITINE,* on the other hand is synthesized by our body from the amino acids *LYSINE and METHIONINE. VITAMIN B3*

# GLOBAL ATHLETES BIBLE

*(NIACIN), B6 (PYRIDOXINE), IRON and VITAMIN C* are all necessary for this conversion to occur successfully. In our own experimental use we have found both to be highly effective, and it is a good idea to include all the foregoing nutritional supplements/vitamins in your athletic ergogenic package.

In terms of performance *L-CARNITINE* is highly essential in the utilization of fatty acids for energy. Experimentally, *L-CARNITINE'S* ability to improve athletic performance and health has been well documented. All indications are that this close cousin of amino acids (but not classified as such), is a substance that transports the fatty acids across the mitachondrial membranes which constitute the power house of our cells. This is actually the place where nutrients are converted into energy. In this way, it controls increases in your body's fat stores that could inhibit optimum performance. *L-CARNITINE* is of considerable value to athletes engaged in all areas of sports. Aside from *CARNITINE'S* many benefits in terms of optimizing health and athletic performance, its attractive feature is also its lack of toxicity. It is an extremely safe ergogenic substance and can yield considerable results in a properly designed exercise program. It is also an excellent weight control/reduction nutrient if utilized as such. In this way, *L-CARNITINE* is currently being used more regularly by many athletes, including ourselves. As a point of caution, *do not* use its D- or DL- forms.

Generally found in meat and some dairy products, *L-CARNITINE* is also involved with our body's dispersal of excess calories. Within our body it is synthesized in the kidneys and liver, with the latter playing a key role in both carbohydrate and fat metabolism, as mentioned earlier. Similar to amino acids, the effect of *ALL B VITAMINS* is synergistic. When discussing the production of energy, it is impossible not to make mention of *VITAMIN B1*. Found abundantly in cereal grains, beans, kidney, etc., this vitamin participates closely in the transformation of glucose into either energy or fat. Without adequate supply of this nutrient, we can easily see that glucose may not be readily converted into energy, thereby adversely effecting performance. *THIAMINE (B1)*, is also known as the "Morale Vitamin" for its particular effect on the nervous system and brain cells. Consequently, it is an essential nutrient for athletic mental energy in the form of quickness and clarity. It is also a critical ingredient in the metabolism of carbohydrate diets. *THIAMINE* deficiency often manifests itself in sluggishness and even depression.

Essentially, all B vitamins are concerned with the proper utilization and absorption of nutrients and the production of energy. As such, they are vital to every cell function in the body. Thus, the *more athletic a person ie., the more functional and developed your muscles, the larger your need for this family of vitamins.* Easily destroyed by food-processing, cooking, caffiene, alcohol etc., supplementary *VITAMIN B1* is essential to the lifestyle of the contemporary athlete. Best intergrated with other *B-COMPLEX* formulas and the *ANTISTRESS ACIDS (PANTOTHENIC and FOLIC),* we recommend 1/2 gram on a daily basis for maintenance.

In medical experiments, *NIACIN* has been found to inhibit fat synthesis in the liver and as such, constitutes an effective aid in combating serum cholestorol and the various fat-cholestoral-protein complexes (LDL< VLDL) which are closely linked to cardiovascular disease and forms of cancer.

# GLOBAL ATHLETES BIBLE

*NIACIN* is also a nutrient beneficial to the mind. It calms the mind naturally. Pellegra, dementia and other schizophrenic symptoms are *VITAMIN B3 or NIACIN* deficiency deseases. *NIACIN* being rather acidic, taking an antacid agent with it usually recommended. For full effect *NIACIN* should be ingested with meals, and there are also sufficient studies to show that its consumption of up to 1,000 mg daily is quite safe and harmless in normal individuals! We suggest that this dosage is quite appropriate and beneficial to hard training athletes. Being necessary for the synthesis of sex hormones, *NIACIN* is also becoming quite well known for its more exotic uses. Taken approximately 30 minutes before an intimate encounter, *NIACIN,* according to some eminent authorities on this subject, *can enhance sexual pleasure and intensify orgasm!* Thus, apart from its medical and therapeutic uses, *NIACIN* may well be the choice recreational nutrient of the future. Note however, that very large doses of *NIACIN*, can cause nausea, and even lead to hyperglycemia.

When discussing the prevention of fat accumulation in the liver in the context of performance, one cannot ignore *LYSINE*, which is also an essential amino acid upon which most body growth factors are dependent. Found in dairy products, *LYSINE* is an essential nutrient, well-known for its ability to release insulin as well as stimulate growth hormone *(GH)*. In combination experiments *LYSINE/ARGININE* have been known to stimulate a far larger *GH* release than either one administered individually; but the corresponding increase in insulin levels should also be monitored. *LYSINE* at any rate is the amino acid which nourishes the blood and bolsters our immune system.

In terms of athletic performance, chronic fatigue, poor recovery rate and lack of concentration, may constitute symptoms of LYSINE deficiency. Chemically related to *ARGININE and ORNITHINE, LYSINE* is less costly than both and is widely used in products that purport to release growth hormone. Such claims should of course be closely monitored as their formulations are more questionable than not. This however, should not detract from supplementary nutrient *LYSINE'S* partnership with the co-enzyme structure of *BIOTIN* which is also essential for the metabolism of fats, carbohydrates, and proteins, and usually included in most *B-COMPLEX* supplements. *BIOTIN*, (also essential for the biosynthesis of folic and pantothenic acid), deficiency manifests itself in muscular pain and lack of appetite and energy. *LYSINE* will compete with *ARGININE* and *ORNITHINE* for transport across the blood-brain barrier, a fact that any administration of *LYSINE* should be cognizant of.

All said, *L-LYSINE* plays a critical part in assisting the biosynthesis of the growth hormone releasing amino acids *ORNITHINE and ARGININE.* A high dosage of *LYSINE* does tend to upset the stomach, although it is a very essential nutrient in the quest of maintaining a high standard of health and fitness. Strenous exertion, athletics, stress, and exercise, all increase the need for these nutrients way more than what is considered a "required level" by the RDA.

Relevant in this respect, is also the essential amino acid nutrient *METHIONINE*. This sulphur-containing essential amino-acid aids in the cleansing process of the liver and kidneys as well as repressing cholestoral deposits and atherosclerosis. *SULPHUR* of course, promotes the maintenance of oxygen balance, is an integral part of tissue building amino acids and works in tandem with the *B COMPLEX VITAMINS*. *METHIONINE* is critical in the liver's manufacture of *LECITHIN*. Contrary to *LYSINE, METHIONINE* does not compete with the other amino acids for transport across the blood barrier and thus can be taken with the well known GH releasing amino acids ie., L-Dopa, Tryptophan, Arginine, and Ornithine. *METHIONINE* also has antioxidant qualities and provides good protection against the free radicals engendered by exercise and other thermogenic nutrients, and as such, is bound to be an amino acid of choice among athletes of the endurance sports. By converting *METHIONINE and LYSINE* our body is capable of producing *L-CARNITINE,* providing of course that the former amino acids are adequately available in our diet. In experimental researches, *CHOLESTORAL* deposits have been linked to *METHIONINE* deficiency.

In order for our bodies to metabolize *METHIONINE* properly and effectively, nutritionists recommend appropriate supplies of *VITAMIN B6*. A daily supplementary dosage of about *1 gram* is recommended for active healthy adults who are free from psychotic tendencies. If the latter case is present, this amino acid may worsen the symptoms and may even compound them with depression. Therefore, use this ergogenic nutrient with caution.

It is also important to note here that there is a high degree of interchangeability between *METHIONINE and CYSTEINE*, the latter being the only other abundant amino acid containing sulphur. Sulphur, is of course essential in the formation of coenzyme A and tourine in our bodies. Eggs, onions and garlic etc., contain high levels of dietary *CYSTEINE*. Pure supplementary *CYSTEINE* is especially effective in combating the effects of free radicals, and in the regeneration of the DNA-RNA components of our cells. Adequate supplies of *CYSTEINE* could considerably forestall aging and the onset of assorted degenerative diseases. It is also a perfect antioxidant for the contemporary polluted environment and lifestyle. It is very important to take adequate doses of *VITAMINS B1 and C* to enhance the effectiveness of supplementary *CYSTEINE* and prevent its oxidization.

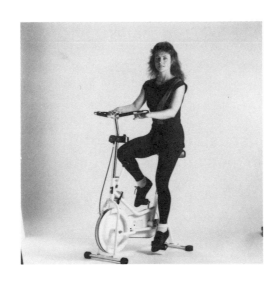

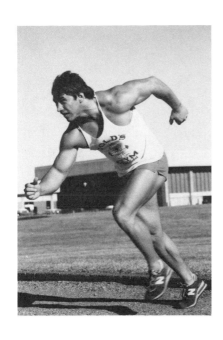

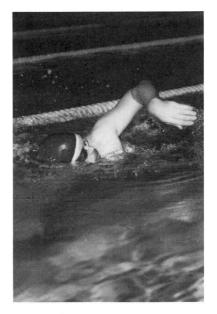

## *THE PROTEIN-AMINO ACID LINK*

### *PROTEIN*

It is very important that all people should obtain adequate amounts of protein in their daily diet, especially athletes who subject their body to intense workouts must nourish their bodies with sufficient amount of quality protein. It is a scientific fact that the need for dietary protein is greatly increased during stressful and physically demanding periods. Scientific nutritional planning requires the balancing of various proteins in order to supply the body with adequate amounts of all the essential amino acids. When consumed, protein is immediatley broken down or hydrolized into its amino acid components. Our bodies can naturally synthesize some of it its amino acids, while those it cannot sufficiently synthesize are known as "essential amino acids". These must consequently be supplied in our diet in order to rebuild our bodies vital tissues and cell structures. Again, if any amino acid is amiss, protein synthesis will not be effective.

To be sure, proteins have a wide variety of functions. There are *contractile proteins* in skeletal muscles such as *ACTIN and MYOSIN* and there are *collagen proteins* that hold our bones and connective tissues together. *COLLAGEN* is the most common protein found in our bodies and *VITAMIN C* is required for its synthesis. What is identified in the body as *COLLAGEN,* is nutritionally speaking, organic silica. Our body synthesizes organic silica into calcium to feed our skeletal development and rejuvenate us at the cellular level. This was the observation of Dr. L. Kervan, who educated the world about the importance of silica.

The role of *VITAMIN C* is also very versatile. Much of it is stored in the adrenal gland, through which it is secreted in stressful situations in the form of *epinephrine* and *norepinephrine.* This conversion however, presupposes the existence of the essential amino acid *L-PHENYLALANINE* in our diet. Also, with its influence on the release of hormone *THYROXINE* from our thyroid glands, it intimately influences our metabolic rate. It is also a key fighter against carcinogens, and collaborates with other amino acids in the making of *COLLAGEN.* As a whole, it is vital to our physical and mental integrity and well being.  Conceived in this way, all the necessary mineral-vitamins and amino acid supplies must be in the bloodstream simultaneously and in proper proportion to efficiently proceed with the bio-chemical demands of tissue synthesis, repair, growth, and ultimately, strength and performance.

From the standpoint of athletic performance, *PROTEINS* provide nutrients for muscular contractions, hasten what is known as the recovery process and build even more contractile muscle tissue for increasing strength, size and recovery etc. This dynamic cycle of muscle tissue production (anabolic) and break down (catabolic), known as protein metabolism, is an ongoing process and is dependant on the large doses of protein nutrients present in our bodies.  Thus, the protein content of our body is constantly undergoing anabolic synthesis and breakdown.

Protein nourishes the entire framework of our body and is a component of our cell, all the ten trillion cells of our body.  Beginning from our skin, right down to our enzymes and hormones, we are protein.  Ninety-five percent of our hemoglobin molecule is protein! In performance terms, hemoglobin, or our red blood flow carries oxygen by chemically combining with it from the lungs to the tissues, and transports carbon dioxide back to the lungs. Our very genes constitute a particular kind of protein. Next to water, is it is the most available substance in our body. Thus, in Greek *"protos"*, which is the origin of the word protein, it means *"first"*.

Nutritionally speaking, amino acids are the chemical units of which proteins are made. Daily digestion breaks down the proteins into their constituent amino acids, which in turn proceed to recreate the thousands of enzymes necessary for digestion. *LIMITING AMINO ACID* is the name given to the most deficient essential amino acid in our bodies.

In brief, protein is an excellent muscle building food, whose primary function relates to the growth, maintenance and repair of muscle tissue. Proteins in our body tissues are in constant motion in this dynamic motion of tissue production and break down, a principle which our daily diet must take into consideration. Simply put, the body constantly uses up nutrients for growth and maintenance irregardless of the supply. If our body finds itself deficient of protein, it simply takes apart existing body proteins in order to gain access to the necessary amino acids. Athletic protein deficiencey manifests itself in poor muscle tone and posture, tissue degeneration, and considerably lowered immunity to injury, disease etc. More relevant to exercise for example, muscle comprises approximately 40% of our bodyweight using about 40% of our energy even at rest. Muscle, it must be remembered, is always an active tissue, and requires a great deal of protein to function at its optimum capacity.

From the standpoint of athletic performance and nutrition, these facts cannot be understated, as recent experiments tend to support our position, that athletes, or physically active people, in most cases, do require quality protein in their diet more so than inactive individuals. The former, simply subject their bodies to more physically demanding activites. To our way of thinking, the more severe the activity the greater the need for protein. The body operates best when the supply and proportion of nutrients is adequate. It follows then, that for people who train hard to achieve their athletic objectives, the recommended daily protein allowance is probably insufficient and in need of state-of-the-art supplementation, as the wear and tear element is much higher in the lifestyle of athletes. Medical evidence also suggests that the need for protein will be greatly increased during periods of extended heavy work load, stress, injury and infection. It is in this context that the dietary supplemention of protein in the form of amino acids, has of late attracted considerable attention from athletes and nutritionists alike.

The interior workings of protein in the ongoing transformation of the athlete's biochemistry, and ultimately performance, are rather subtle and proceed in a complex fashion. During contraction of the muscle tissues, for example, the key chemical and protein molecules which are responsible for all muscle contraction are formed *(CREATINE, MYOSINE, and ACTIN.)* respectively. As a point of illustration, *GLYCINE* is the key amino acid involved in the metabolism of muscle cell. Its natural conversion into *CREATINE* enables it to store phosphates in the muscle and retain adequate amount of *ATP* (adenosine triphosphate) which in turn constitutes the energy plant for all muscle contraction. Muscle fatigue thus calls for increases in this amino acid. This nonessential amino acid

# GLOBAL ATHLETES BIBLE

*GLYCINE,* is now used by physicians in the treatment of muscular dystrophy and it has also been found useful in the improvement of pituitary gland function and treatment of hypoglycemia. Perhaps an over simplified explanation of protein's role or need in muscle chemistry, but the point of note here is the key role it plays in the development and quality of our skeletal muscles, tissues, and structural intregity. It follows then, that sufficient protein must be available to achieve quality gains in size, strength and performance, whatever the athletic endeavour. Every athlete wants to gain quality muscles and burn fat. Bodybuilders and other power athletes have repeatedly reported greater gains with the use of proper amino acid supplementation to complement their workouts. Athletically speaking, the quality and amounts of amino acids in a protein determine its nutritive and performance value. In short, you need *ALL* the amino acids in your dietary and supplementary protein if you are going to have an opportunity to build and rebuild quality muscles that grow and perform when called upon. Throughout these discussions, remember that the effects of all the amino acids is synergistic.

# GLOBAL ATHLETES BIBLE

Our experience in this respect, has been parallel to theirs, and thus, why protein supplementation constitutes a great part of our program, both for ourselves and our students when appropriate. We emphasize this latter point since protein requirements do vary widely among different types of athletes, depending on their genetics, sex, size, activity, and lifestyle. In other words the strength, type and intensity of the activity will determine an athlete's protein need, in the form of necessary amino acids. Protein, thus conceived, is indeed the "building block" for power performance and athletic strength. Protein nourishes our every cell. We always recommend a balanced daily intake of amino acids from protein sources, including dessicated liver, tofu and whey. With the connective tissues and fat removed, liver constitutes an excellent source of protein. The latter two have also proved to be easily assimilable and digestible nutrient sources of protein. When purchasing protein formulas, the well-informed athlete should always read about how the formula was put together. What are the amino acids of concern? Are there any digestive enzymes? If so, which? How are they proportioned? Is there a balance? what is the bacteria count etc.? In other words at the very least, read the labels carefully and make critical use of your information on amino acids.

As a main source of energy food, protein assumes a secondary role to carbohydrates and fats. In terms of performance only about half the calories of protein can be converted to energy per se. In other words, protein is not a significant energy source.

The processes in this dynamic cycle of *PROTEIN METABOLISM* are induced by the rapid mobilization of our body's structural proteins, which are fueled by *AMINO ACIDS*. Proteins are then broken down into individual or short chains of amino acids (peptide bonds) by the digestive process. Peptide bond refers to the chemical link between one amino acid to another. The majority of biochemical reactions require amino acids in their free forms rather than in peptides.

Thus, chemically speaking amino acids may function in long chains known as proteins, in short sequences called peptides, or may function alone. There are really hundreds of proteins, with each being a different combination of amino acids. Upon digestion, dietary proteins are split, and enter the blood stream into their constituent amino acids. To adequately perform their biological functions all essential amino acids must be in the bloodstream simultaneously. The "secret" here is to have a balanced diet of natural foods that provide adequate amino acids. Strictly speaking, the importance of protein for our purposes, is not in itself, but in the amino acid properties of its contents. At this point, a digression to the functions of amino acids is in order.

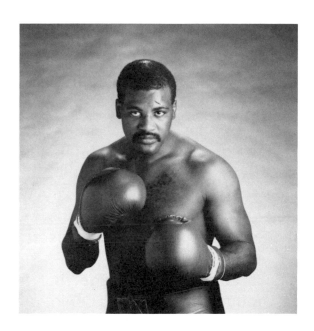

## *IMPORTANCE OF AMINO ACIDS*

In terms of chemistry, amino acids are composed of hydrogen, carbon, oxygen, nitrogen and at times sulphur. Amino acids are also the precursors of neurotransmitters, enzyme cofactors etc.

Commonly known as *the building blocks of life*, amino acids are the basic components of proteins, absolutely essential for life and the body's primary source of nitrogen. Athletically speaking, the degree of nitrogen loss depends of course upon the severity and duration of the exercise, stress or injury. It has been conclusively proven that *LEUCINE, VALINE, and ISOLEUCINE* provide about 70% of the free nitrogen to the body. *Nitrogen*, is of course vital for the body in order for muscle growth and protein bio-systhesis to occur successfully. Science tells us that approximately 75% of the body's dry weight is composed of chains of amino acids known as protein. Protein in turn, is composed of 16% nitrogen.

It is also common knowledge that the body requires around 22 amino acids in a specific pattern to produce human proteins. During stressful exercise or training a great deal of this *AMINO ACID* pool provides the energy required to support protein synthesis in the functions of our organs and our skeletal system. In terms of performance, the energy production takes place through the oxidation of what are known as the *BRANCHED CHAINED* amino acids *(BCAA'S)* inside the muscle tissue, and through the *GLUCOSE ALANINE* cycle. When under acute physical or emotional stress, our amino acid reserves in the body are mobilized and converted by the liver to glucose *(blood sugar)*. To provide energy for these increased physiological demands *LEUCINE (BCAA)* is rapidly oxidized and synthesized into glucose, particularly enhancing the athletes endurance capacity, while simultaneously freeing the appropriate amino acids to proceed with their task of protein synthesis. In this way, exercise recreates a pool of amino-acids to be consumed for muscular hypertrophy (growth). If sufficient quantities of the *BCAA'S* are not present however, the loss of muscle tissue will occur, and performance will suffer considerably, since the body will be forced to break down and borrow proteins for energy use. From this angle, it is not hard to discern that the proper *PROTEIN* types and needs of athletes must be designed very carefully. Particularly in times of stress, the proteins derived from the so called *Branched Chained Amino Acids (BCAA's)* such as *LEUCINE, ISOLEUCINE and VALINE,* are set in motion as major regulators for the body's physical and emotional energy output, thus sparing protein for other relevant biochemcial functions. Their deficiency is certain to compromise athletic performance, the healing process and tension tolerance in daily living. The exact requirements of protein depends of course on the volume and intensity of the training and the particular type of sport practiced. Amino acid supplements and protein powder products in this respect have proven invaluable and more easily assimilable than "knife and fork" proteins. These natural products are designed for optimal food restoration and synthesis, and have proved to be very effective athletic aids.

The dynamics of the process may be outlined as follows: Of the 22 amino acids, 12 are classified as non-essential, which the body produces from the remaining ten, (or nine depending on which source you consult), that are classified as essential, because the body cannot synthesize them. Hence they must be extracted from food sources that are referred to as complete proteins (they include all the esential amino acids). It is common knowledge now that all the essential amino acids must be present simultaneously and in proper proportions for the body to utilize its protein supply properly. The dietary protein quality of a food is rated accordingly. The essential amino-acids in complete protein food sources may not necessarily be in proper proportion to one another, thus ultimately, it is their *assimilability ratio* which provides nutritionists the basis for rating complete proteins. In short, your daily diet should aim at providing you with complete proteins, or a combination of complementary protein sources which amount to the relevant quality.

In terms of understanding diets for example, it is important to know that eggs meet the existing requirements of a complete protein. In terms of the digestive process they rate a high level of assimilability, estimated at 96%, thereby setting the standard for what is known as *PER* or the *PROTEIN EFFICIENCY RATINGS* used by nutritionists. In brief then, the protein content of nutrients can be determined by the presence or absence of the essential amino acids in proper proportions.

A single gram of protein equals approximately 4 calories, the same amount of calories as carbohydrates. Conceived in terms of activity, non-athletic persons, or an inactive athlete should consume 1/2 gram per pound of body weight, while the active male athlete, to our way of thinking should take in about a gram per pound of body weight. That is a gram of complete protein, or about 33% of the daily caloric needs. The female athlete should consume one gram per kilogram of body weight. Again, caloric needs vary from individual to individual, but evidently, the athletic individual in training needs significantly more protein than the sedentary individual. Seen from the point of view of obtaining higher levels of physical tolerance, efficiency, and performance, the quantity and combination of foods and needs of athletes are different from non athletes. Different athletes also vary in their needs, depending of course, on their bio-chemisty and chosen athletic endeavours. This is where nutritional counselling assumes great importance. Anything less than an adequate supply of protein in an athlete's diet can cause performance setbacks, if not serious health problems. By the same token, *overconsumption of protein can result in even more serious health hazards,* including ketosis and kidney damage.

Certain qualities and considerations of protein can impeded or upgrade the *PER* tremendously, thus effecting performance. Briefly, for example, milk (a popular beverage among athletes), has a known assimilability ratio anywhere from 60% to 90%. Pasteurized milk has the lowest *PER* and raw milk the highest. Eggs when combined with milk make for real complete protein, upgrading the *PER* of the diet considerably. Incidentally, dairy products constitute good sources of *LYSINE, TRYPTOPHAN, ARGININE, and METHIONINE.* That is all the amino acids necessary for the formation of tissue protein. These are useful diet tips for hard training athletes, who use protein supplement drinks. For those who are concerned with the cholestoral content of eggs, nutritionists recommend the product *LECITHIN* (a cholestoral absorbent) which is available at most health food stores. Fish (also a popular food among athletes), has a low fat content, is easiest to assimulate and constitutes a substantial protein source. It has a high biological value. Poultry-chicken etc., also rank high in terms of assimilability. They contain top quality protein and are very rich in *ARGININE*. On the other side of spectrum, beef and lamb are the most difficult to assimilate. The fat factor and content in animal meat can also cause indigestion for several hours. When cooked, it's chemistry is altered placing undue stress on the liver and kidney functions essentially overloading them, possibly to toxic levels. We do not conceive animal meat as particularly ergogenic and in fact recommend its drastic reduction and combination with the appropriate pure nutrient supplements. Better athletic results are emminent.

To avoid the pitfalls associated with animal meat and fat, many competitive athletes, including ourselves, rely more and more on first-class protein nutrient supplements in the form of free form amino acid mixtures to achieve peak performance levels. This is not be read as an encouragement for the indescrimenate ingestion of supplements. 60% of our protein should still come from *PLANT* sources and should be combined and supplemented with the individual athlete's needs and deficiencies in mind. Administered in this way, they will have a high biological and performance value. Remember, excessive reliance on supplements can have detrimental effects as well. Thus, amino acids are not only the digestive products of protein, but also the building blocks of protein.

## *PROTEIN IN ATHLETIC PERFORMANCE*

Next to water, we have stated that protein is the most plentiful substance in the body. Briefly protein is one of the most important ingredients for the maintenance of good health and vitality. It is a major source of building material for growth and development of muscles, blood, skin, hair, nails and internal organs including the heart and the brain. As such, proteins are indispensable to all living cells in our body. Uniquely too, proteins contain nitrogen. The protein content of our body is in constant motion. The human body must obtain nitrogen from protein sources as it cannot utilize the nitrogen *(N2)* which is found in the air. In daily activity nitrogen is constantly emitted from the body through skin, hair, perspiration, waste etc., and replaced through dietary protein or supplementation. Thus, nutritionally speaking everybody needs a minimum amount of daily dietary protein to make nitrogen available for tissue rebuilding etc. Athletes need more nitrogen supply to meet the challenges of daily training, or the body will rob its own tissue protein as a source for the missing amino acids.

Simply put, the RDA *(recommmended daily allowance)* for protein is set according to a positive nitrogen balance. Positive nitrogen balance is when we take in more protein than we lose. Negative nitrogen balance on the other hand refers to the state described above, where we use more protein than is retained, a condition not suitable to building and maintaining performance at any level.

Many world class athletes and coaches believe that in order to gain muscle strength and improve performance we must be in positve nitrogen balance or training time may be totally wasted.

Thus, the current RDA of one gram per 2.2 pounds of bodyweight, falls far below the requirements of an athlete in training.

# GLOBAL ATHLETES BIBLE

Contemporary sports nutrition points to the direction that athletes do indeed require more protein than the average inactive person, and are relying more and more on protein formulas and supplementations. Bodybuilders and competitive athletes striving to increase muscle mass and maintain peak performance standards may require more yet, in our observation. Consequently, a training athlete will learn how to balance his body's protein needs, with his glycogen (carbohydrate), and daily caloric needs. Aside from our strong belief in supplementation, we try to impart the following information to our students.

First and foremost, as an athlete you have to carefully select the nutrients that give you more or less complete proteins. If there is a missing or disproportionate essential amino acid, then there exists a limiting factor in the entire dynamic of protein synthesis. In your coordinations, you have to project 100% assimilability when you select your protein diet. Eggs, milk, tofu, and whey for instance, have very high assimilability ratings because more of their amino acids are used by the body than in any other food. That is, they rate as complete proteins. Through their inclusion in his/her diet, an athlete can adequately meet the challenges o his/her training and daily living.

As a point of warning, however, *DO NOT* stuff yourself with protein. Calories beyond those required to maintain bodyweight will almost always be added in the form of bodyfat. Excess protein that we cannot use as building blocks, repair material or energy reserves, is broken down by the liver into fat and glucose and is stored as body fat. *EXCESS PROTEIN CAN MAKE YOU RETAIN WEIGHT (BODYFAT).* A condition that reduces performance significantly.

Thus far twenty two amino acids used by the human body have been conclusively identified. Here is a list of *"essential" and "non essential"* amino acids for your convenience.

# GLOBAL ATHLETES BIBLE

## CLASSIFICATION OF AMINO ACIDS

| ESSENTIAL | NON ESSENTIAL |
|---|---|
| L-Histidine | L-Alanine |
| L-Iso Leucine | L-Arginine |
| L-Lysine | L-Aspartate |
| L-Methionine | L-Cysteine |
| L-Ornithine | L-Cystine |
| L-Phenylalanine | L-Glutamate |
| L-Leucine | L-Glutamine |
| L-Threonine | L-Glycine |
| L-Tryptophan | L-Proline |
| L-Valine | L-Aspargine |
| | L-Serine |
| | L-Tyrosine |

*L-ARGININE AND L-HISTIDINE* are semi-essential, necessary for normal growth and developement but not required for the maintenance of nitrogen balance.

Chemically speaking, amino acids come in either *D or L form.* The two forms are considered *"mirror images"* of each other, as opposed to identical, and only the L forms can link together to form protein chains. Consequently, natural amino acids are for the most part in L form. Some D amino acids on the other hand, such as *D-METHIONINE and D-PHENYLALANINE,* do have unique properties that can be beneficial to some individuals suffering acute physical injury and pain.

In this context, a 50%-50% mix of *L-PHENYLALANINE* and its mirror image, *D-PHENYLALANINE* has produced *DL-PHENYLALANINE (DLPA)*, which has proven extremely encouraging in combating acute physical trauma, through the manipulation of our body's innate ability to control chronic pain. Experimentally, *DLPA* has brought relief to patients who have suffered for many years and its athletic uses are also at a promising experimental stage.

*L-PHENYLALANINE* on the other hand, is of late, making some remarkable inroads into the athletic world. This essential amino acid is concentrated in most high protein foods, such as meats, milk, and cheese, which have traditionally constituted the staple diets of athletes. Chemically, *L-PHENYLALANINE* is the natural converter of the neurotransmitters *NOREPINEPHRINE (NE)* and *DOPAMINE*, which dispatch signals between the brain and nerve cells. Note however, that *VITAMIN C and B6* are essential for the conversion process to occur successfully and efficiently.

Unlike the other chemical stimulants

# GLOBAL ATHLETES BIBLE

such as *AMPHETAMINES* etc., which actually deplete our *NORADRENALINE* (the brains version of adrenalin), *PHENYLALANINE* is converted into *NORADRENALINE* and released naturally into our system. *L-PHENYLALANINE*, when ingested as a single amino acid, releases *THYROXINE,* which in turn stimulates mental clarity and retention as well as enhancing our energy levels markedly. Scientists have also found types of depression and drug addictions rather responsive to *PHENYLALANINE and THYROXINE* therapy.

Because *PHENYLALANINE* is one of these amino acids that has to compete with other protein nutrients for access into our brain, nutritionists suggest that it is best ingested on an empty stomach. Dosage has to conform to individual needs and characteristics, depending on many variables. Personally however, we have found *one gram* of supplementary *PHENYLALANINE* first thing in the morning, to be a very effective stimulant and facilitator for training when the pressure is on. If this dosage should prove too high for you, behavioral changes such as excessive irritability and aggression etc., will soon indicate  that you should reduce your intake.

*People with cardiac problems and a history of hypertension should exercise great caution with this nutrient.*

From the point of view of athletic performance then, natural nutrients and amino acid supplementation ensures that the body's necessary functions are carried out to their optimum potential. They've been known to aid in:

A. The reduction of body fat and blood sugar levels.*(CARNITINE, ARGININE, NIACIN)*

B. Cardio-vascular endurance ie. The heart and the network of blood vessels. *(SELENIUM, NIACIN, GAMMA ORYZONOL, INOSINE, VITAMIN E, etc.)*

C. Repairing and regenerating broken down muscle tissues. *(LYSINE, GREEN-LIPPED MUSSELS, SILICA, VITAMIN C)*.

D. Increasing muscle size, mass` and strength by triggering the body's mechanism to release growth hormones, this is particularly the use with the singles (freeform). Similar to the anabolic effect of steroids which will be discussed later. *(L-ARGININE, L-ORNITHINE, L-LYSINE)*.

E. Cleaning out the digestive and intestinal transport tracts. *(L-THREONINE)*

F.   Reversal of nervous and personality disorders.

G.   Regeneration of the cells of the kidney and liver and relieving arthritic rheumatic disorders *(METHIONINE, GREEN-LIPPED MUSSEL)*.

H.   Combat against free radical damage, and the effects of smoking and alcohol. *(CYSTEINE, ORNITHINE ARGININE, VITAMIN'S E and C, G.O, etc.)*

I.   The detoxification process of athletes. *(TYROSINE, TRYPTOPHAN)*.

J. Warding off chronic fatigue and depression.*(PHENYLALANINE, TYROSINE)*

K.   Immunization against diseases. *(ARGININE, ORNITHINE, CYSTEINE, VITAMIN C )*.

L. Enhancement of intelligence. *(CHOLINE and VITAMIN B5, or VALINE)*

M.   Controlling anxiety, stress, and anger. *(VITAMIN B6 and C, TRYPTOPHAN)*

The various benefits described above of course depend on the availability of adequate amounts of amino acids and vitamins in specific proportions.   In terms of athletic performance, all the essential amino acids must be available in the diet along with the appropriate precursors for the synthesis of the non-essential ones, to provide all the 22 amino acids necessary for the body's anabolic and catabolic demands.

Although it is wise to start out with low dosages, in our experience, the optimal dosage allowed on the labels is quite harmless to healthy individuals, providing the right cofactors are present. Amino acids in the blood stream are known to exist at about 30-40 grams for three to four hours.

Authorities who have written at great length on this subject caution that isolated amino acids should not be taken at the same time as completes. Unless there is approximately two hours between the two, the effects of the single will be negated in the ensuing competition to cross the blood-brain barrier. At this point an illustration of this dynamics is appropriate.

Despite the prevailing confiçt of information, it's pretty clear that *L-ARGININE and L-ORNITHINE are GROWTH HORMONE RELEASERS WHEN APPLIED COMPETENTLY* and in the proper *ratio of 2:1*, and at the right time and dosage. They have proven popular among athletes of late, as natural and potent anabolic hormone stimulants. It is recommended that they be ingested either in the morning on first awakening or in the evening. It is a physiological fact the *GH* is naturally secreted approximately 90 minutes after the onset of sleep, and again just before awakening, in the morning. Thus, *GH* releasers appear to have more effect when administered in the evening. The specific applications however are rather tricky and warrants some qualifiers. It is imperative that everybody work up to the proposed dosages gradually. *ORNITHINE and particularely ARGININE* have been invaluable supplements in our own athletic endeavours. *ORNITHINE'S* use is still at a rather experimental stage among athletes. *ARGININE* when taken in large doses has demonstrated promising results as a natural *GH* releasing nutrient.

If you decide to take them at bedtime for instance, they should be administered with *approximately one gram of L- TRYPTOPHAN* in order to counteract the tendancy of insomnia that could be brought about by their combination. Used in this way allow less than an hour for the effects of *TRYPTOPHAN* to be felt. It is very effective in reducing what is known as sleep onset latency and used with excellent results as a natural relaxer by athletes. It is also documented that taking a complementary carbohydrate snack with *TRYPTOPHAN* will increase the amount that enters your brain, ie., its crossing of the blood-brain barrier. Also unlike other sedatives and tranquilizers on the market, this essential nutrient does not hamper coordination, affect our judgement and reaction time. Note that *VITAMINS C and B6* are essential for the effective conversion of *TRYPTOPHAN* into the natural brain chemical and neurotransmitter, *SEROTONIN*. The latter is associated with neurons that control body temperature, mood, and sleep.

In this context, *PYRIDOXINE (VITAMIN B6)*, is extremely vital in that it plays an important role in the metabolism of carbs, fats, and protein, and in their transport within our skeletal system. *PYRIDOXINE* is particularly essential to amino acid and carbohydrate metabolism. It also aids in the conversion of *TRYPTOPHAN to NIACIN*. Among other things, its antioxidant properties are absolutely important to all athletes and all health conscious individuals. This vitamin also functions as a natural diuretic and regulates the antiaging nucleic acids. *PYRIDOXINE* requirements are determined by the overall diet and supplemental amino acid intake, and the athlete's needs, training habits, physical condition, etc. All things considered *500 mg* of supplemental *PYRIDOXINE* in your *daily* nutritional package will help maintain an efficient sodium/potassium balance, as well as a healthy nervous system and efficient brain function.

The effects of the single amino acids vary from one individual to the other. *L-ARGININE*, for example, could cause viral infections to flare up in some people. In this case, and if administered approximately sixty minutes after the combination, *L-LYSINE* helps suppress any viral reaction that may arise. *L-LYSINE* is an essential amino acid that plays a key role in our body's growth and repair mechanism. It is a critical amino acid in the process of protein metabolism. Performance wise, it is necessary for the proper utilization of the fatty acids required for energy production. Experiments in Europe have also demonstrated *LYSINE'S* particular anabolic properties when combined with *ARGININE*. It is also known to compete with *ARGININE* and *ORNITHINE* for transport across the blood-brain barrier and should not be taken together with the former.   Thus, the suggested sixty-minute interval.   In terms of performance, it is directly involved in the production of *CARNITINE,* a chemical substance also required for the utilization of fatty acids in energy production.   *LYSINE* is also known to promote better concentration. In the extreme case where the athlete harbours herpes simplex, the *L-ARGININE* will cause its symptoms to flare up, in just about every instance.   This is the side effect of this amino acid so to speak.   Of late, *LYSINE* has been found effective in the combat against herpes.  As a whole, *LYSINE* supplementation improves the protein quality of nutrients and is strongly recommended.

Perhaps it's due to their widespread commercial use, most recent discussions on *GH* releasing amino acids starts from *L-ARGININE and L-ORNTHINE.*   In a cyclical process, *ARGININE* is constructed from *ORNITHINE* and the latter is released from *ARGININE.*   Fundamentally, *ARGININE* is an essential nutrient available in animals while *ORNITHINE* is classified as non essential.  The latter has twice the biological activity and is consequently twice as effective as the former.   In practical application 1 gram of

*ORHITHINE* releases twice as much *GH* as a gram of *ARGININE*. *ARGININE* in its own right is a highly important nutrient. Seminal fluids for example are known to contain 80% *ARGININE!* Its supplementation can conceivably increase sperm count. *ARGININE* is a building block for proteins, and essential for the normal functions of the pituitary gland. It is however, the remarkable fat loss and muscle building effect of *ARGININE* supplementation that has of late emerged as a subject of much favorable practical and theoretical research. This is not really surprising, along with *PHENYLALANINE, ORNITHINE* is also a neurochemical nutrient necessary for the secretion and synthesis of human growth hormone.

In order to convert *ARGININE and/or ORNITHINE* for *GH* secretion purposes, additional supplementation of the amino acids *LYSINE* and *TRYPTOPHAN, and VITAMINS B6 and C* are also recommended. Both *ARGININE and ORNITHINE* amino acids nutrients have low toxicity, with the former providing better experimental results in the athletic quest of building maximum muscles with minimum fat. Chemically, *ORNITHINE* helps insulin function as an anabolic hormone. Certain food sources are relatively high in *ARGININE* content (dairy, chicken) etc., but for athletic purposes their consumption is much less effective than the pure nutrient supplements. For best effect, the recommendation is that they are best taken in the right proportion, on an empty stomach and approximately an hour before exercise. We are certain to hear more about the athletic benefits of *ORNITHINE and ARGININE*, in the near future. The dosages recommended on the manufacturer's bottles are very safe and athletes in training condition can in fact slowly increase their dosage depending on their specific needs and physical condition.

It is ultimately up to the athlete to arrive at an approximate combination of amino acid supplements, dosages and modifications, depending on his/her particular needs. For maximum benefit from the amino acid supplementation, a well balanced vitamin and mineral program is essential. Applied knowledgeably, the athlete's performance can benefit significantly from the optimal nutrition, supplements, and physical exercise routines he/she have designed for him or herself. What we would primarily like to underline here is that individual differences be considered in all nutritional issues. Everybody needs a necessary level of minerals and vitamins to function adequately. The minimum *RDA* is basically a figure arrived at from the point of view of preventing nutrient deficiency among the population as a whole. As such, it varies from country to country, and takes daily survival as it's point of reference. In the final analysis, it is more expedient and temporary than scientific.

Athletes on the other hand, must look at nutritional requirements with a view towards their long range impact, and take optimum health and performance as their frame of reference. Consequently, it is not hard to see that athletic endeavours require higher levels of nutrient than those calulated by official *RDA'S,* both in quality and quantity. Certainly no significant athletic record can be shattered by administration motivated *RDA* dietary guidelines!

Nutritionally speaking, the value of many foods are usaually limited by the absence of one or more essential amino acids. In this case they should be complimented with supplements rich in the amino acid of concern. For maximum effect, always check how much *pure amino acid* you are getting. As a serious athlete, your calculations must start here.

## *INJURY FIGHTERS*

For injuries that often occur among athletes, *MUSCLE FLEX* has lately proved a reliable and effective nutrient compound. Originally used for rheumatic and arthritic conditions, this supplemental nutrient derived from green-lipped mussel (an edible shellfish cultivated in New Zealand ), has proven valuable in combating muscle stiffness and commonly occuring tendon pulls. This so called "injury fighter" nutrient is rich in balanced amino acids, enzymes, minerals etc. Mussel has also demonstrated considerable abilites in restoring muscle elasticity, by successfully promoting tissue repair and maintenance.

The effect of this nutrient on athletic performance is not unlike that of shock absorbers on vehicles. By providing a water bed type of coating around our cells, it gives our skeletal system the necessary protection and extra resilience it needs to perform optimally. Whether *AQUALITE or SEATONE,* all mussel based supplementary nutrients have similar protective functions for athletes.

Dosages of these injury fighters should be administered at approximately 1 1/2 to 3 grams daily at the onset of injury, and progressivley decreased with the decline in pain and discomfort. People with a history of high blood pressure should exercise caution with this supplementary nutrient. Among the supplementary products involved in the healing process of athletic injuries ie., fractures, tendon pulls, etc, the herbal *BF & C FORMULA* is also highly effective and recommendable.

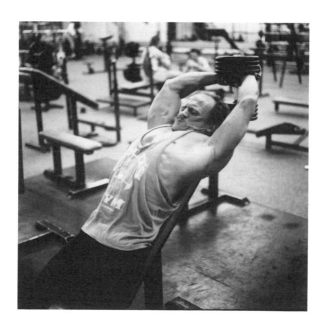

# GLOBAL ATHLETES BIBLE

## *STEROIDS*

Many world-class, and *too many* aspiring athletes and bodybuilders are attracted to a group of drugs known as *ANDROGENIC-ANABOLIC STEROIDS,* because they believe that it builds up the requisite strength and muscles to give them an advantage on their competition. The *"juice"* as it is known among users, has been on the sports scene since the fifties, but its prevalence these days is causing legitimate concern and alarm among athletes, coaches, professsional sports officials, and the medical profession. Even the *IFBB* (International Federation of Bodybuilders), that bastion of steroids, is taking some serious steps to eradicate steroids from the bodybuilding sport. It also happens to be a requirement for the olympic status that it seeks.

Once the domain of veterinarians, strength and speed athletes, the widespread use of steroids as they are more commonly known is a more recent phenomenon. Like their track and field colleagues, other athletes have also taken to steroid use of late, in the belief that steroids make it possible to build more muscle, train harder and recover faster. All happen to be vital ingredients in the attainment of peak performance standards. Female athletes and bodybuilders in search for increased performance have also taken to steroid substances of late, with devastating results and little or no competitive advantage in the long run. In this fashionable way, the market is fast reaching down to the younger generation of athletes who are rather ignorant and/or misinformed about the health hazards and psychological problems associated with androgenic-anabolic steroid use and abuse. On the other hand they are highly mesmerized by it's magic appeals and promises. Driven by their blind athletic ambitions or certain deep seated psychological needs, young athletes simply and conveniently ignore the risks involved, until they are too late into the vicious steroid cycles. Ever more powerful and expensive European imports are also surfacing on the North American market. Although steroids are powerful chemical substances regulated under the *Food and Drug Act*, officially available only on perscription and banned in every professional sport, national and international competitions, their growing demand and casual *"underground"* availability raises some serious medical and ethical questions. In short, official position, notwithstanding what is known as *"institutional steroid use"* is widespread and rather incidious in todays sports world, both amateur and professional. This is what has brought the issue of drug testing to the foreground.

In Canada, it is not illegal to possess these drugs, while trafficing them is a criminal offence, on the same level as narcotics. Under these circumstances, the illicit dealers of these substances are experiencing a profitable boom and their territory is rapidly expanding right down to the highschool and neighbourhood gyms. Today steroids are as readily available to athletes, in the same fashion as cocaine and heroin are to junkies ie., secretly and at a price. It is in this context, that this chapter will proceed to explore this steroid dilemma prevalent today. It is meant to inform and educate on the hazards of steroid consumption.

Our knowledge in this area comes both from theoretical and practical sources, that include our own brief experimental steroid use and that of our associates. *Dangerous side effects from steroids are a scientific fact today*, and we categorically don't endorse or recommend their use by any athlete. There can no longer be any pretenses on this issue. Today, the question is actually approached in terms of minimizing the well known health hazard associated with steroid use. From our point of view this attitude can no longer be justified. Health threatening anabolics and ergogenics must be roundly condemned, and supplemented with the appropriate natural alternatives that do not stunt growing adolescents, possibly for life. Athletes can't afford risking the destruction of their health to remain competitive. This appears to be contrary to the athletic spirit, as we see it.

Thus, while we believe in, and wholeheartedly recommend natural supplementation, we strongly warn and discourage steroid use to potential users who have of late approached us on this subject. Steroid use can no longer be considered a valuable training aid, particularly in the face of contemporary enlightening scientific athletic and nutritional breakthroughs.

What then are these substances exactly? Androgenic-anabolic steroids are functionally and chemically related to the male sex hormone testosterone (this is what *androgenic* means) and are used to accelerate weight gain and growth (this is what *anabolic* means). Thus, when people speak of steroids in athletics today, they are talking about possible increases in size and strength *(anabolic)*, and the production of secondary male sex characteristics such as muscularity, deeper voice tones, facial hair, aggressive behavior, etc., *(androgenic)*.

In terms of familiarity with steroid chemistry this is a rather important basic information, since there is no such thing as a purely anabolic or androgenic steroid. All steroids have various proportions of androgenic and anabolic properties, and come in what is known as an *anabolic/androgenic ratio*, and a rather misleading therapeutic index. By common consensus the *therapeutic index* is calculated by dividing the anabolic ratio by the androgenic ratio. Derived from animal research however, the various anabolic/androgenic ratios and therapeutic indexes are at best inexact and vague indications. Inexact, because they do not really tell us the exact effects of the particular steroids on athlete's living in the real competitive world of sports. This is rather unfortunate, since steroid use, or abuse, which is more often the case, adversely effects the athletes personality as a whole. Mild paranoia to more serious psychopathic disorders of the mind have been linked to steroid abuse. Rats in captive laboratory experiments hardly have to suffer the consequences of their misguided actions and decisions for many years to come. This is a unique human trait, and bears some reconsideration.

The more *serious side effects of steroids are irreversible,* even after the suspension of steroid use. Nevertheless, presented in this way, and as potent ergogenic devices, there are currently a variety of steroids on the market promising different effects on our musculo-skeletal and growth systems. It is also rather obvious that no two people will react the same way to steroids. That is, steroid chemistry manifests itself differently in different people, depending on their use and personal bio-chemical make up. Unqualified experimentation could have hazardous consequences on the user's physical and mental condition.

In terms of improving athletic

performance, the different steroids are defined and classified by what they imply to deliver. Some like *DINABOL* are regarded to exceed in gaining size and strength, while others like *MAXIBOLIN* excell in tissue building and toning functions. Still others, like *METHYLTESTOSTERONE* activate aggressive impulses both in the gym/field and outside. Steroid induced aggression seriously impairs your sense of judgement. As far as the underground literature on this product is concerned, "be prepared to be one hell of a mean son of a bitch," who hates everyone and everything else when you are on this *"juice"*! The psychological implications of this profile should not escape us. It primarily promotes and glorifies anti-social behaviour.

There are also steroids for keeping muscle mass, like the popular German import *PRIMABOLIN-S*. Yet others like *BOLASTERONE* promise to decrease recovery time as well as increase mental alertness and reaction time. Some are deemed to reduce bodyfat and the French import *PARABOLIN* is said to give your physique a hard appearance within about a week. The anabolic/ergogenic varieties and combinations are endless. There is also the Italian steroid *ESICLENE* whose particular reputation rests on making the specifically injected muscle area (deltoids, biceps, quadriceps,) grow. With reference to this particular product, what occurs upon injection is really a swell, brought about by chemical irritation and divertion of blood into the area. It is a temporary *"fix"*. Thus, whereas the emphasis differs, this family of drugs as a whole promises to promote and boost physical developement and athletic prowess in a relatively short period of time.

Lest the above presentation should be translated as a shopping list for steroids, it must be pointed out that without the appropriate know-how, dosage, and " stacks", these are simply product names used for illustrative purposes and are insignificant in themselves. Referring to the actual application of steroids, stacking must be designed according to what the athlete is trying to accomplish, and constitutes a very complex business requiring blood chemistry profiles etc. Dosage ranges and the way they are administered involves what users refer to as cycling their steroid intake. In brief, a steroid "cycle" consists in using several drugs in various combinations for various periods. A cycle typically lasts anywhere between six to eight weeks.

Steroids generally come in two forms, that may be classified as orals and injectables. Buccal tablets which can be dissolved under the tongue, are also available. As far as steroid chemistry goes, their real difference does not lie in the origins of application, ie., either orally or injected intra-muscularly, but in the ways our bodies assimilate, hydrolize, and synthesize them throughout our musculo-skeletal system, and their biochemical reaction within our system.

In this respect, both kinds of steroid application have their specific qualities and charcteristics. *Contrary to popular belief, the injectable steroids are NOT more toxic and stronger than orals,* except in very few cases. The reasons are related to what is known as the *"17 ALPHA AKYLATED PROCESS"* undergone by the orals, in order to make them more conducive to absorption by our system. That is to say, the chemical modification known by this name is clinically responsible for their toxic levels.

By common consent among the experts on this subject, the popular *ANADROL-50* is definately the most toxic towards our liver and aromatizes at a higher rate than all the others. This concept of the aromatization of steroids simply calculates the rate of conversion of the steroid to female hormonal characteristics or estrogen, by our bodies, and also introduces the issue of side-effects long associated with steroids. To compound the problem, sooner or later, ie., depending on dosage, all high androgenic steroids aromatize to a certain degree, except possibly for *PARABOLAN and FINAJECT*. Simply put, the body produces excessive female hormones to stabilize hormonal imbalance, hence aromatizaton will result. The somewhat puffy and bloated physique, often accompanied with testicular shrinkage, acne, and advancing female breast characteristics (gynecomastia), are symptomatic of this process. In most cases, the weight gain on the scale is symptomatic of water retention. In female users, the symptoms manifest themselves in pronounced masculine traits, deeper voice tones, facial hair, agressiveness, enlargement of the clitoris, and irregularities in the reproductive system. In the face of these reactions to the male hormones, female users must therefore take extra cautions with the *anabolic/androgenic ratio* of their intake. High androgenic steroids even at what are considered "normal" dosages, are absolutely hazardous to the female athletes structural and mental integrity. Aromatization, as well as high dosage and ill informed use may advance many of the side effects associated with continual steroid abuse. Symptoms are precipitated by the existing hormonal imbalance in the body, and can have serious consequences, both physical and mental. The evidence is everywhere and simply too obvious to ignore.

On the question of dosage, where a lot of grossly incorrect and superficial ideas are rampant, a few words are in order.

The affinity of the partricular steroid to the receptor sites in our musclo-skeletal system more or less determines the dosage classification of the steroid in question. That is to say, some steroids come in very high dosages ie., 50 mg tablets, while others come in 2 mg tablets. The high dosage, indicates the particular steroids poor affinity for the receptor sites in our bodies, while the low dosage indicates the opposite ie., it takes a lot less of the drug to get to the receptors. Since the steroid receptors in our system can only absorb a certain amount of the drug, in case of excessive use, the receptors simply shut off, pouring the excess into our system and causing what is known as the "spillover" effect. This process needless to say, enhances the various side-effects associated with steroid abuse. Ultimately, high blood pressure, liver dysfunction, distorted facial lines, elbows, feet, and foreheads, are some of the more revealing physical characteristics of steroid abuse. These are grave health problems. Thus, there is absolutely no doubt in our mind that the long term use of steroids significantly affects the structural integrity of our musculo-skeletal system as a whole, ultimately defeating the purpose of our regular exercise and nutritional program.

Because of the aura of taboo and illegality associated with this family of drugs, most users are forced to depend on the pushers of these substances for instruction, dosage, and use program. If one is convinced he/she must use steroids at all, this is a risky way to go. The dealers credentials in this respect are usually quite deficient, and their motives questionable. We have personally heard of many critical mistakes in quality, dosages and suggested timing of intake, which if undetected could have resulted in serious hormonal imbalances, despite the apparent few pounds of gain, strength, and overall euphoria experienced by the novice user. In most cases steroids merely mask fatigue and injury factors, which immediately rebound after the suspension of use. The complex personality distortions generally referred to as *"steroid psychosis"* will also undergo modificatioins with type, time-span and quality of steroid use. The athlete's chances of being one of the athletes who are dependent upon steroids both physically and mentally is quite high, while his/her chances of achieving their desired athletic objectives without the proven side effects, are rather negligible.

As far as the dealers of steroids go, their profit motive must always be kept in the back of your mind. The supply for a cycle of steroids can cost anywhere between $200.00 and $2,000.00, with extremely lucrative profit margins! Once into a cycle and the influences are felt, most people do not have the mental fortitude to get off them, and accept the consequences of apparent weight loss and mental leveling. They no longer feel strong, big, and aggressive. Most complain of lost libido. Self esteem appears significantly reduced. As a matter of fact, there is a feeling that they are shrinking, losing control of their training, and hence unable to meet the challenges of daily living. Withdrawl from steroid use is a serious business. Until otherwise enlightened, educated, and nutritionally fortified, many aspiring athletes will inevitably constitute the captive market for steroid dealers and their products. The cost to users are quite varied and manifold. For example, steroid users are strongly advised to use various anti-estrogen agents in their stacks in order to eliminate the effects of aromatization. For this purpose *NOLVADEX* is the most popular and the recommended dose is one tablet a day at a cost of about $2 a pill!

Aside from the prohibitive cost factors, there is really neither proof nor consensus on their real effectiveness. There is really no conclusive evidence that steroids really achieve the task they were originally intended for. They do certainly maximize physical output, but they do have many proven detrimental effects, while the gains may well be mostly the result of heavy training.

*Nolvadex* certainly does not actually block estrogen but only inhibits the already elevated levels of estrogen, and if the dosage is not precise, it may actually increase the estrogen levels already in existence! To get around this phenomenon, steroid users are usually recommended to use another anti-aromatization agent like *PRO-VIRAN* in their stacks. Again, this steroid substance may or may not live up to their promises, depending on the individual bio-chemistry, level of training, nutrients, quality of cycling, etc. By now it should not be too hard to discern the remarkable hazards associated with cumulative steroid use and experimentation.

Steroids are transported to the receptor sites in the cells by two plasma carrier proteins, affecting virtually every cell in the body. Upon ingestion, the orals are assimilated into the musculo-skeletal system and synthesized, (or hydrolized as the experts refer to the process), by the liver, in approximately 24 hours, not counting the residual steroids, which are detectable under clinical conditions. Different steroids have different lifespans in our system. Once hydrolized the steroids disperse throughout the steroid receptors into the muscle and bone cells.

# GLOBAL ATHLETES BIBLE

Injectable steroids follow a similar procedure, although they are hydrolized by the liver much more gradually. With few fast acting (acetate) exceptions, experts estimate it takes the injectables anywhere up to three days to be thoroughly hydrolized. The water based injectables are considerably faster acting than the oil based drugs which are in the majority. The water based variety passes through the system much faster than the oil based products which are stored longer in the body. Some athletes feel this makes them safer and less detectable for drug testing purposes. The injectables with the oil base generally linger in the body for much longer, anywhere from one to three weeks, whatever the rate of hydrolization. It takes oil based injectables only about three days. The choices are personal and sport specific, but the consequences health threatening and social, and this is where the ethical aspects come into play.

In our own experience steroids generally promise more than they deliver, and harbour unacceptable risk factors that athletes can no longer afford to ignore in their single minded quest for athletic excellence. Once we started looking more closely into this area, we read everything we could on the subject and learned a lot of important facts we didn't bother to familiarize ourselves with earlier.

The answer, we think, lies in the proper understanding of the functions of growth hormone. Medical science has discovered ways to trigger the body's release of this hormone naturally, the specifics will be described in the following chapter.

Suffice it to say at this point, that *GH* is in abundant supply in growing bodies and can be increased through natural methods of supplementation to full advantage. Thus, it is grossly incorrect and shortsighted, to provide steroids to athletes who haven't stopped growing and have ample supply of *GH* in their own bodies. *Ultimately, steroids will compromise and retard the athlete's physical developement.* The alternatives on the other hand will stimulate your natural gains and protect your health. It is the way of the future.

# GLOBAL ATHLETES BIBLE

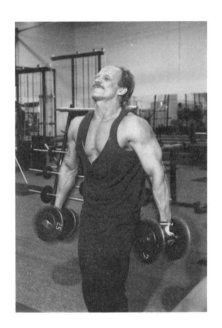

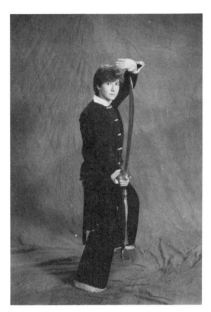

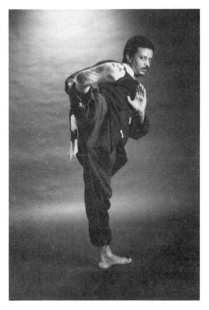

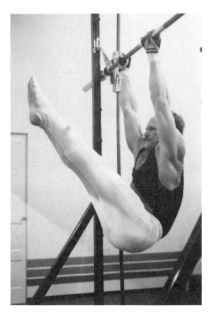

# GLOBAL ATHLETES BIBLE

## *THE STEROID ALTERNATIVE*

While the steroid experiment amounts to nothing other than a risky chemical experiment with human engineering, the system of training we have ellaborated on in these pages, may be conceived in terms of a scientific and naturalistic human para-physiological manipulation. In our system natural nutrients and supplements factors play a major role in the achievement and maintenance of peak athletic performance levels. Regular coordinated training, adequate rest, the dietary manipulation of athletes, when balanced and scientifically approached, constitute the bare foundation of the Global system , under whose inspiration we have been operating.

In order to ellaborate on this system's characteristics a little deeper however, let us clarify a few concepts at this point. It is this system that provided a critical point of reference for our own development as athletes and performance nutrition consultants. Above all, this system is personality and sport specific. That is, it seeks to improve and enhance the ability of athletes to perform in their own chosen sport.

# GLOBAL ATHLETES BIBLE

It is also consistent with contemporary lifestyles and scientific developments.

In application, this system avoids the extremes of fasting for a certain number of hours, and does not pander to trendy diets and fitness fashions. It's success depends, on the applications of scientific bio-chemical laws, in the coordination of nutrient substances and vitamin-mineral complexes known to stimulate and enhance the attributes required for safe optimal athletic performance.

Thus, in short, our system focuses on enlisting the known *natural anabolic* (*GH* stimulants) and *ergogenic* (energy enhancing), nutritional aids, in the service of athletic excellence. Of late, many elite athletes, have incorporated a variety of this approach in their training preparations for Olympic level competitions. In principle, this approach is anchored in our understanding of *GH* releasing nutrients, and is definately the way of training for the future athlete. It has been our experience with this approach, that when properly applied, excellent natural gains in overall performance can be stimulated in all serious athletes. Major changes in body composition can be apparent within approximately two months. Being free of the various health-threatening side-effects associated with anabolic/androgenic steroids, this approach is also consistent with the temprament of the times, and coincides with our practices, and present commitments as athletes.

The guiding principle of this method of training, consists of the use of specific, individualized, dietary and training supplements, to release the body's own anabolic and neurological resources (biological, hormonal, cellular, enzymatic) etc., without introducing potentially dangerous pharmacological substances into or system. Steroids, amphetamines and cocaine, may actually cheat athletes from the full realizaton of their natural potential, while robbing the other competitors of savouring the fruits of their natural athletic prowess. On the personal level, their long term consumption will typically result in lowered vital energy and disaster.

Since experimental scientists have discovered that increased *GH* levels can be manipulated by appropriate nutritional supplementation, the use of nutrient *GH* releasers has become widespread in the sports world, and among health conscious fitness enthusiasts as a whole. In paricular, the fat loss and muscle gain benefits of the *GH* releasing nutrients, was well received among athletes who easily recognized the ergogenic potentials involved in such a chemistry. Early experimental successes with athletes, and in particular female bodybuilders, have firmly established such *GH* releasing nutrients as *ARGININGE, ORNITHINE, LYSINE, and PHENYLALANINE* as the choice athletic nutrients of the eighties and beyond.

What is known as *GH,* or growth hormone, is located in the brain's hypothalmus, and secreted through our pituitary gland, which has been identified as the precise hormone responsible for regulating the fat loss and muscle growth function of our body. In the final analysis, the hypothalmus regulates all the hormonal or endocrine activity in the human body, and as such, constitutes the centre of interest for our approach to performance nutrition.

Scientists inform us that everybody is naturally endowed with abundant supply of *GH* in the body. It is absolutely essential for protein synthesis, tissue repair, muscle growth, and maturity, etc. It also plays an important role in the mechanism of our immune system. During adolescence, it plays a critical role in metabolizing body fat into muscles and energy, for our maturing years as healthy teenagers. It is also known that human *GH* release progressively declines, and further drops with aging, virtually stopping when we approach our fifties. It's precise relationship to the aging mechanism is the subject of considerable research, but it is known that by using natural nutrients that activate *G H* levels, it is possible to remarkably reverse the aging process, in the context of fat loss, muscle-building, skin tone, flexibility, etc. *G H* in our bodies is naturally secreted during exercise, sleep, stress, etc., and being indigenous to the body, it can be triggered and manipulated through safe, natural nutrient amino acid supplements, which are for the most part, available in any health food store, without perscription.

The application and use of these nutrients however, is rather complex, experimental in nature, and involves specialized nutritional knowledge and ingenuity. Simply ingesting supplements will not result in any benefits whatsoever; In other words more supplementation does not result in elevated *GH* functions in our bodies. The quality, timing and overall diet of the athlete are determining factors. For anyone enjoying a medium to heavy exercise program regularely however, it is essential that the special *GH* releasing effects of certain amino acids and other nutritional supplements be put to proper use and in the proper perspective.

We certainly do not know everything there is to know about administering *GH* releasers because it is still at the experimental stage. There are certain fundamentals however, which every serious athlete must be expected to know. We try to explain the bare scientific basis of our recommendations for every *GH* releaser that we have had the opportunity to familiarize ourselves, and experiment with.

From the point of view of athletic performance *GH* releasing supplements come in several forms. However, the most relevant and accessible ones for our purposes are available in health food stores, must be orally ingested and require no perscription whatsoever.

Decades of research on the part of scientists all over the world is lately discovering a host of nutrients that may empower the human body with remarkable *GH* releasing potentials well into its advanced years. With their advent, nutritional science is truly undergoing some revolutionary changes, which every serious and health conscious athlete should follow up on. From the point of view of competition, it is no longer possible to maintain an edge without proper attention to these nutrients, whose use is fast becoming very popular among athletes and health conscious fitness enthusiasts all over the world. We think this new phenomenon promises some excellent opportunites for the natural alternative method of maximizing physical and mental performance.

Following, is an introductory presentation of the most widely used and highly regarded athletic nutrient compounds which influence the release of the human growth hormone mechanism without any known adverse effects on the integrity of our skeletal system and organs.

In this context the athletic community has welcomed the rice extract *GAMMA-ORYZONOL* as a potent ergogenic substance particularly as an anti-oxidant and hormonal regulator. This white powder derivative of rice, was first discovered by a Japanese research scientist some three decades ago, but has only recently come to the attention of the western world on such a wide scale. Through its effect on the hypothalmus, preliminary experiments suggest that *"GO"* is capable of stimulating anabolic as well as fat dissolvig properties in our bloodstream. As an effective antioxidant, it also helps as a free radical scavenger, thereby enhancing the body's production of efficient energy much on the same order as *SELENIUM and VITAMIN E.* In fact, it is mostly prepared in combination with the latter and in a *ratio of 1:5 (20 mg of GO with 100 IU of Vitamin E)* for best results.

Its qualities may be especially attractive to athletes involved in endurance oriented sports with heavy aerobic contents. Again, taking all other relevant factors into consideration, a supplemental dosage of approximately *10 mg daily* should give a good practical indication of how it works for your personally. The dosage can be raised when appropriate.

The organic compound *INOSINE* has also responded to the athletes call for increased gains in performance. *INOSINE'S* particular ability to maintain and replenish the universal energy molecule *ATP* has come to the attention of the sports world. Research has shown that depletion of *ADENOSINE TRIPHOSPHATE* results in diminished oxygen supply and muscle fatigue, similar to the type experienced by glycogen burnout. The nutritional supplement *INOSINE* has been found to penetrate both cardiac and skeletal muscle in replenishing and stimulation of *ATP* production at the cellular level. As such, it has been hailed as an *ATP* precursor par excellence. Technically speaking *INOSINE* promotes the production of chemicals essential in the transport of oxygen molecules within our system. By a complex series of chemical interactions, *INOSINE* can allow for more intense workouts and performance levels by boosting cardiac output and endurance.

Another supplemental nutrient which is making its appearances on the athletic scene is also from Japan, where it has been widely used for over a decade. Known as *CO-ENZYME Q10*, it has been used by millions of Japanese with cardiovascular and energy concerns. With its impact on the cells, *CO-ENZYME Q10* helps to elevate and regulate oxygen in our skeletal system and is vital for energy output, immune system efficiency, and in general cellular health.

Taken according to the directions on the label, supplemental *CO-ENZYME Q10* is a pure, natural and safe way to restore to our body what advancing age, diseases and stress progressively withold from us and interfere with. At any rate American scientists and sports nutritionists are reacting favorably to the qualities of *CO-ENZYME Q10*. In our own experiments a dosage of 50 mg daily has proven rather safe.

Some other nutrients and plants that have long been known for their ability to rejuvenate and heal the human body, have also shown remarkable athletic benefits. Although presently, they may not be used as such, these natural nutrients like *GINSENG, FO TI TENG, HO SHOU WU, and BEE POLLEN,* can be extremely useful in tonifying our vital organs, restoring and increasing energy, vigor, and stamina, in the most natural way possible. While the classical tradition of martial arts thrived on these potent oriental ergogenic substances, a contemporary martial artist like Mohammed Ali has claimed that he used *BEE POLLEN* granules successfully all during his championship years of training and fighting. Many other olympic stars and athletes have also made similar uses of *SEAWEED* and other herbal remedies like *SKULLCAP*, in their training diets. This coincides with the growing movement among professional athletes to avoid the *health-threatening* and *potentially dangerous* family of drugs known as *steroids*, in favor of the natural alternatives.

In the herbal world, varieties of *GINSENG* are considered to be the most potent tonics in their effect on the well-being and efficiency of the entire body. *GINSENG'S* ability as a cardiac tonic and energy stimulant is almost legendary. People in the west have only recently learned to appreciate the potent ergogenic and powerful healing properties of this oriental root plant. It is interesting in this context, that *GINSENG* also has considerable amount of *GERMANIUM* in its composition.

For anyone who wants to maximize athletic potential naturally, it is worth their while to study organic *GERMANIUM'S* properties. Developed in combination with the amino acid *L-GLUTATHIANE* and other vitamins, the benefits of *GERMANIUM* are presently available to athletes as *GE OXY-132.* Simply put, this *GERMANIUM* combination works with our oxygen transport mechanism to boost oxygenation, immune functions, and performance. Through it's unique electron transfer properties, *GERMANIUM* works with oxygen to maximize cellular energy and tissue function throughout our body.

Not surprisingly, the richest amount of organic *GERMANIUM* were found in nutrients that have a history of solutory effects on health and energy ie, garlic, aloe vera, comfrey, mushrooms etc. Research is sure to fully unravel the ergogenic qualities of these nutrients and others like *WILD YAM,* in the near future and present them in formulae that are effective and easily assimilable to the human body. The possibilites are truly limitless.

Of late, a host of presumably ergogenic substances are emerging on the market, with some amounting to nothing more than very costly iron/amino acid supplements. *CYTOCHROME C* and possibly *ALPHA-KETOGLUTARATE* may belong to this category, *DIMETHYLGLYCINE or DMG,* and *WHEAT GERM OIL/OCTOCOSONOL* both have high contents of *VITAMIN E* and are the current rage of nutrients. Some athletes have approved of their endurance-promoting qualities, while others have voiced reservations about these products. Ultimately, time, research, and experimentation will prove the true efficacy of all these supplemental nutrients in athletic performance. Meanwhile, based on the available information, we will continue to use a variety of experimental approaches and combinations to enhance our scope of knowledge in this important area.

In the final analysis, the mysteries inherent in mankinds physical culture have existed for centuries and will only be resolved by constant scientific experimentation. *We are still destined to be what we eat!*

# GLOBAL ATHLETES BIBLE

## GLOBAL OUTSTANDING ACHIEVEMENT AWARD

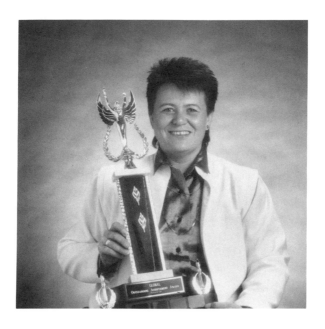

### LINDA COHEN

Global Health is proud to take this opportunity to introduce to our readers Ms. Linda Cohen, 36, from Edmonton. A nominee for the 1986 Vanier Award, the current Multiple Sclerosis, or *MS Person of the Year,* and holder of our *Global Outstanding Achievement Award* for 1986; Linda is an exceptionally talented and courageous wheelchair athlete, with a most worthy cause to pursue.

Confined to a wheelchair for the last 8

years of her young life, Linda is nevertheless, the first woman in our province to complete a 3,000 kilometre wheelchair marathon throughout Alberta, in order to raise funds for Multiple Sclerosis research and treatment. This dreaded, tissue destroying disease of the brain and spinal cord, for which medical science has found no known cause or cure, affects approximately 50,000 Canadians. It is our opinion that they could have never found a more able and committed spokesperson.

Indeed, Canada is considered a high risk area for MS, which is known to be more prevelent in the latitudes furthest from the equator. As such, her odyssey and goals should really concern us all.

We at Global Health, have accepted the challenge and are totally committed to helping this dynamic lady organize and train for a super-marathon, that will take her wheeling from Mexico to Edmonton, at some time during the 1988-89 period. This trip projected at approximately 4,500 kilometres, holds some new challenges as well as opportunites for Linda and MS in general. Linda's optimism is almost infectious, but her athletic prowess, stamina and endurance are sure to be tested to the maximum.

On our part, we will pay particular attention to Linda's training and supplemental needs, in the hope of fortifying her body adequately for the upcoming challenge. The task has only just begun, and we hope to be "wheeling" with her until she achieves her goals.

# GLOBAL ATHLETES BIBLE

## *ACKNOWLEDGEMENTS*

We wish to extend particular gratitude to the helmsman David Nyholt, for encouraging us to build this book in the first place, and for generously sharing his facilities and wisdom.

Noel Zinger's sharp eyes and excellent suggestions have also been priceless in the photographic illustrations of this work.

## *POSTSCRIPT*

After extensive research and experimentation with nutritional supplementation, the following products have in our opinion demonstrated consistently high quality delivery. We would not hesitate to recommend their use to any adult who intends to pursue a fitness lifestyle and utilize the nutritional principles outlined in these pages.

## Recommended
## Global Hi-Tech
## Supplements

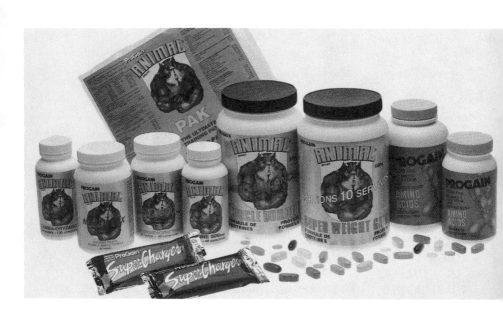

# UNIPRO
## PERFORMANCE NUTRITION

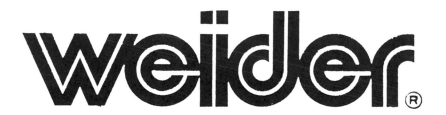

# GLOBAL ATHLETES BIBLE

## BIBLIOGRAPHICAL NOTES

*DR. ABRAVANEL'S BODY TYPE PROGAM FOR HEALTH, FITNESS AND NUTRITION* - Elliot D. Abravanel/Elizabeth King, *The Bantan Book,* 1985.

*ADDITIVE ALERT* - Linda R. Pim, *Polution Probe Foundation, 1986.*

*AMINO ACIDS BOOK* - Carlson Wade, *Pivot Original Health Books, 1985.*

*I. ASIMOV-THE HUMAN BODY AND THE HUMAN BRAIN-* Isaac Asimov, *Bonanza Books.*

*DR. ATKINS' SUPER ENERGY DIET* - Dr. R. Atkins/S. Linde., *Boutam Edition, Feb 1978.*

*DR. BERGER'S IMMUNE POWER DIET* - Stuart Berger, M.D., *A Signet Book 1983.*

*BODY DEFENSES* - Marilyn Dunlop, *Irvin Publishing Inc. 1987.*

*THE CALCIUM BIBLE* - Patricia Hausman, M.S., *Warner Books, 1985.*

*CALORIES AND CARBOHYDRATES* - Barbara Kraus, *New American Library NY, 1985.*

*CARNITINE: THE VITAMIN BT PHENOMENON* - Brian Leibovitz M.S., *Dell Publishing, 1984.*

*DESIGN YOUR OWN VITAMIN AND MINERAL PROGRAM* - Shari Lieberman M.A., R.D., / Nancy Bruning, *Doubleday, 1987.*

# GLOBAL ATHLETES BIBLE

*DIGESTIVE ENZYMES* - Jeffrey Bland, *Keats Publishing, Inc., New Canaan, Connecticut. 1983.*

*EAT TO WIN* - Dr. Robert Haas, *Signet Classic, Feb. 1985.*

*FIGHTING DEPRESSION* - Harvey M. Ross, *Larchmant Books, 1975.*

*FIT FOR LIFE* - Harvey & Marilyn Diamond, *Warner Books, Inc. 1985., N.Y.*

*FOOD FOR CHAMPIONS* - Ned Baynard/Chris Quilter, *Berkley Books, New York, 1984.*

*HEADACHE CONTROL WITHOUT DRUGS* - Andrew Wm. Serada, MD., FRCP (c) Neurology, *Amarantine Press, 1987.*

*LET'S EAT RIGHT TO KEEP FIT* - Adelle Davis, *Harcourt Brace Jovanavich, Inc, 1954, 1970.*

*LET'S STAY HEALTHY* - Adelle Davis, *A Signet Book, 1983.*

*THE LIFE EXTENSION COMPANION* - Durk Pearson/Sandy Shaw, *Warner Books, Inc. 1984.*

*THE LIFE EXTENSION WEIGHT PROGRAM* - Durk Pearson/ Sandy Shaw, *Doubleday & Company, Inc. 1986.*

*LIVING HEALTH* - Harvey & Marilyn Diamond, *Warner Books, Inc. 1985 N.Y.*

# GLOBAL ATHLETES BIBLE

*THE NATURAL & DRUGLESS WAY FOR BETTER HEALTH* - M.O. Garten, D.C., *Parker Publishing Co.Inc., 1969.*

*NEW CONCEPTS IN THE PREVENTION AND TREATMENT OF NERVOUS SYSTEM SYMPTOMS AND ILLNESSES* - Andrew Wm. Serada, MD., FRCP., (c) Neurlogy, *Armarantine Presss, 1987.*

*REPS BUILDING MASSIVE MUSCLE* - Robert Kennedy, *Sterling Publishing, 1985.*

*ROCK HARD* - Robert Kennedy, *Warner Books Inc., 1987.*

*SELENIUM AS FOOD & MEDICINE* - Dr. R. A. Passwater, *Keats Publishing, Inc., 1980.*

*VITAMIN BIBLE* - Earl Mindell, *Warner Books, Inc., N.Y., 1981.*

*VITAMIN E* - Herbert Bailey, *ARC Books, Inc. N.Y. 1971.*

*VITAMIN & HERB GUIDE* - *Global Health Publication, 1987.*

*VITAMINS, MINERALS & OTHER SUPPLEMENTS* - Carlson Wade, *Pivot Original Health Books, 1972, 1983.*

*ULTIMATE MUSCLE MASS* - *An OEM publishing, Edited by Daniel Duchaine.*